A MIDSUMMER
NIGHT'S SCREAM

from Paperback Trade Inn
145 East Fourteen Mile Rd
Clawson, MI 48017
2012 (248) 307-0228
Sept.

(handwritten: from Jake, 2012 Sept.)

BARD'S BLOOD #2

A MIDSUMMER NIGHT'S SCREAM

A NOVEL BY DAVID BERGANTINO
BASED ON *A MIDSUMMER NIGHT'S DREAM*
BY WILLIAM SHAKESPEARE

POCKET **STAR** BOOKS
NEW YORK   LONDON   TORONTO   SYDNEY   SINGAPORE

This book is a work of fiction. Names, characters, places and incidents are products of the author's imagination or are used fictitiously. Any resemblance to actual events or locales or persons, living or dead, is entirely coincidental.

An *Original* Publication of POCKET BOOKS

 A Pocket Star Book published by
POCKET BOOKS, a division of Simon & Schuster, Inc.
1230 Avenue of the Americas, New York, NY 10020

Copyright © 2003 by David Bergantino

ISBN: 0-7434-5623-8

First Pocket Books paperback edition August 2003

10 9 8 7 6 5 4 3 2 1

POCKET STAR BOOKS and colophon are registered trademarks of Simon & Schuster, Inc.

Front cover illustration by Jerry Vanderstelt

Manufactured in the United States of America

For information regarding special discounts for bulk purchases, please contact Simon & Schuster Special Sales at 1-800-456-6798 or business@simonandschuster.com.

A MIDSUMMER
NIGHT'S SCREAM

PROLOGUE

The few witnesses to the lights streaking through the sky were either drunk, half asleep or up to some illicit activity in the early morning. Three glowing balls, orange against the milky white cataract of a hazy summer night sky, approached from the west. Much of the ground they passed over were flatlands: undeveloped government property—*seemingly* undeveloped government property—hiding military secrets and a multitude of farms, some of which were themselves fronts for clandestine government installations. But the orange lights ignored these things. They were likewise ignored by the billions of dollars of sensitive equipment pointed skyward. The balls of light had no radar signature, nor were they measurable by any other earthly instrument save the naked eye.

So the soldiers, disguised as restless farmers, ignored the passing lights, figuring the state-of-the-art technology bristling around them would cause a small red light to blink somewhere if anything was truly amiss.

Finally, the bogeys reached an expanse of land where the barns actually housed animals, hay and pitchforks. These actual honest-to-God-and-may-He-bless-America farms soon gave way to a semirural area dotted with trees and houses. Further east, the houses overtook the greenery, save for trees lining streets or sculpturally decorating local parks.

Since it was two-thirty in the morning, the town was mostly dark. Like moths, the glowing objects flew straight for the town's one bright landmark. Halogen lights bathed a water tower, revealing it in all its Midwestern glory. Upon the great tank that overlooked a sprawling college campus was painted a football wearing a gleaming crown. Above the crown were the words *Stratford, Ohio,* and below, *Home of the Globe Monarchs.*

The trio of lights circled the water tower twice and then peeled away after their second pass. Two headed south, to the older, grungier, industrial section of town. The third flew northeast, plunging earthward not far from campus.

In his new apartment, courtesy of Globe University, Professor Ajit Waman sat before a brand-new Ikea desk. His thick body fit snugly in the new, padded Ikea desk chair. The only illumination in the room was from the likewise new desk lamp (Espressivo from Ikea) sitting upon it. The tangle of packing bubbles, Styrofoam padding and strips of plastic straps spread across nearly every inch of floor gave the apartment the appearance of a strange nest or cocoon. Waman ignored the mess. He was used to it.

Up near the ceiling, a vent hummed as the central air redoubled its efforts to keep the summer heat and humidity at bay.

With one hand, he turned over the final page of the lesson plan he had been preparing, while his other hand absently stroked his black hair, ending with a tug at the ponytail that ran between his shoulder blades. Tomorrow would be his first class, and he wanted things to run smoothly.

And it would go smoothly, he assured himself. Those students would learn, summer session or not.

While he turned his plans over in his head, he noticed the room had become brighter. An orange light shone from outside. At first, he thought a helicopter was buzzing the neighborhood, but it made no sound. Glancing through the window, he looked up. A fireball appeared to be falling from the sky. Taking a step back, he watched it fall into frame before his window, but instead of continuing to the ground, it stopped, hovering before him, a globe about the size of a softball, spitting orange sparks that evaporated almost immediately. Soon, it floated like a ghost through the window and entered the apartment. Waman did not speak or move as it approached. It stopped a foot away. At first, it did nothing, bobbing gently in midair, as if observing him. Despite its appearance, it gave off no heat, and it didn't burn its image into Waman's eyes.

Then, noiselessly, it blossomed, sparks cascading from it like a Fourth of July sparkler. Waman took a step back. A figure began to appear from within the lightshower.

Tall and hulking. Horned like the devil. The light soon faded, leaving only the creature. He could see the beast in full now: lips curled back in a snarl over fangs, cloven hooves. The light had given birth to a dark demon.

Without a word, Waman began backing away from the creature. He nearly slipped on the packing materials littering his floor.

With a crack, the desk split in half as the creature stepped through it.

The sound made Waman loose his footing, and he fell, the floor crackling as giant packing bubbles burst underneath him. Pumping his legs, he could find no purchase in the slippery, cushioned floor.

Within two thundering steps of its hooves, the creature was upon him.

1

Summer clung to Lenore like a sumo suit after a championship match. She would have been thankful simply to feel sweaty, rather than coated in hot slime. As she trudged across the Globe campus, she could feel the coverup under her eyes melting away. This July had so far been the hottest on record, and of course the dorms had no air-conditioning. For the past several evenings, she had lain awake on top of her sheets, basting more than sleeping.

Worst of all, the stifling weather was depriving her of the pathetic satisfaction of at least *dreaming* about her unrequited love. And her wilted state would hardly recommend her when she saw the object of her affection in class.

Dimitri Carlton.

Lenore unconsciously clutched her books to her chest as she thought his name, her lips silently forming each syllable. Dimitri had a superhero jaw, with shoulders to match, and a smile full of teeth expensively whitened and straightened.

They had gone out on exactly one date. He'd been sullen to begin with, not much of a conversationalist, but after a few shots of Jägermeister, he'd become a touchy-feely drunk. Later that night he'd touched her in several ways and places no one had ever touched her before, and she'd been smitten. He'd never called her after that, but at least he continued to acknowledge her when they ran into each other on campus and at the bars. And after a few Jägers, if no one else was around, there was always a kiss.

But nothing more. In recent weeks, since he had developed an infatuation for her friend Mia, he barely even acknowledged her presence.

"Oww!" she cried as mascara ran into her eyes. She closed them to avoid further pain as she rummaged through her handbag in search of tissues.

Careful, she thought. *Last time you did this, you superglued your hand to the lining.*

Finally her fingers closed around a soft, plastic-wrapped packet.

Suddenly, there was another hand in her bag. It was rough, like the claw of a giant lizard.

The thought made her scream in terror and pull away. Her heel hit an uneven section of pavement and she nearly fell on her ass, but she steadied herself.

Out of reflex, she dabbed her face quickly with the entire packet of tissues, plastic packaging and all. Her eyes still stung when she opened them, but at least she could see. Mostly.

Lenore let out a surprised squeal.

Before her stood a man with a ragged, matted beard. Shaggy hair framed his face, which was deeply lined and the hue of motor oil. His clothes were a mismatched collection of shreds turned various shades of brown by dirt and probably various bodily fluids. Even his face was stained brown, which made the violet of his irises even more arresting. They would have held her mesmerized had not the stench rising from the man broken the spell. It confirmed what his appearance suggested: He was a vagrant. She had seen him around before, just never up close and personal like this.

His expression seemed to mirror Lenore's terror and confusion, along with a great deal of embarrassment and sadness. He held one of the hair scrunchies that had been in her purse.

"Please. I need money." His voice was as ragged as his appearance. "For some cotton candy."

"Why didn't you just ask . . . what did you say?" Lenore asked, suddenly forgetting her shock, her anger and even her stinging eyes.

The violet-eyed vagrant took a sudden step forward and clutched her shoulder desperately.

"They're here, you know," he croaked at her. His breath was nearly overpowering. "They took Audra last night."

Lenore struggled to pull away, but his grip was firm.

"Hey!" she yelled, more out of surprise than fear. "Let me go!" Then she tried to twist away, but he held her tightly. *Now* she was afraid. "Help! Help!"

"Hey! Get away from her, dude!" she heard someone yell in the distance; a group of burly students had seen the commotion and had started running her way.

Fearful, the homeless man released Lenore.

"I'm sorry," he said, desperation in his voice. "I just need some cotton candy. I just . . ." His voice trailed off, and his violet eyes glazed over for a moment. Then he returned to the present and realized that in moments, the burly students would be upon him. He dashed away around the side of the Science Building and disappeared.

Assuring her saviors that she had not been harmed, Lenore continued to class. In truth, Lenore *was* fine. And though she had been frightened, she was certain he had not intended to hurt her. He had only wanted money.

For cotton candy.

What the hell?

Checking her watch as she entered the Science Building, she found herself with just enough time to touch up her makeup.

In a nearby bathroom, she smeared the quasi-flesh-colored stick under each eye. The face of her best friend, Mia, loomed up in the mirror behind her, interrupting her in the act of blending away her dark circles.

"Hi-eee!" she chirped. The smile she wore evaporated when she saw what Lenore was doing. "Puh. Leaze. You are *not* gussying yourself up for Dimbulb, are you?"

"I'm not!" Lenore said, resuming her blending of coverup with rickety nonchalance. "Not that you care, but as it happens, I was just attacked!"

Mia didn't even look up from the mirror, where she examined her face for faults. Of which there were none.

"What, did Dimbulb wanna ravish you on the Lawn?" she said, lightly pressing a fingertip to her face as if touching up her makeup. She wore none. "I wish Dimbulb would go for you, then maybe he'd give me a break."

Mia stepped back from the mirror to examine her outfit. The look screamed post-punk slacker: black leather mini, lace-fringed tube top and thick-sole boots. The labels within the clothes smugly whispered *rich* post-punk psuedo-slacker.

"No. I'm serious," Lenore said, trying not to compare her relatively frumpy fashions to Mia's. "Some homeless guy. Reached right into my bag when my eyes are closed and took one of my scrunchies."

"Just goes to show you even the homeless can have fashion emergencies." Mia tugged the bottom of her tube top, exposing an extra half-inch of her breasts. "Perfect," she told her reflection.

Lenore turned to her friend angrily. "Mia, I could have been hurt!"

"Oh, sweetie," Mia said, switching to doe-eyed sympathy in an instant. "I'm so sorry." Then her eyes lit up again with her devil girl glow. "Which one was it?"

"Which what?"

"Which homeless guy? Was it Ass-Face? You know, the one-eyed guy who doesn't wear a patch, and the scar tissue makes his eye socket look like an anus?"

Lenore mock-choked in genuine disgust. "No, it wasn't him. It was the guy with purple eyes."

Mia's eyes went wide at this news. "Oh, him! He's my favorite. If you just look in his eyes, you can almost forget he's homeless. Hose him down for, like, a week, wrap him in a Brooks Brothers suit, and he'd be ever so yummy."

"Great. I get attacked, and you get the hots for my attacker. Sounds like a Gerry Springer show: My Best Friend Fell in Love with my Rapist."

This made them both laugh, and any worry over the attack evaporated. Together, Mia and Lenore left the bathroom and headed to class. As she walked, Lenore pulled at her dress so it didn't seem stuck to her like papier-mâché.

"Wow, that near death experience got ya all hot and bothered, didn't it, sweetie?" Mia started to help adjust Lenore's dress as a tease, but Lenore batted her friend's hand away.

"Stop it! It's like a fucking sauna out there. I don't want to go to class looking like a *Night of the Living Dead* extra."

Mia remained unconvinced. "I bet Ole Purple Eyes pawing you was as close as you've come to gettin' some in months. You're like, all Spanish fly and pheromones. You gonna go in there and bop Dimbulb in the head with your club and drag him off by the hair?"

"Stop it, Mia, just stop it!" Tears threatened to well up behind the dam of Lenore's coverup stick. Mia often played at some form of harsh, but now she was just being cruel.

Apparently sensing she had crossed a line, Mia held Lenore back just before the door to their biology class.

"Look, sweetie." Mia softened her voice and cut both the sarcasm and the melodrama. "I love you almost enough to do you myself, if I swung that way." Lenore tried to pull away but had no better luck escaping her friend's grasp than she had her attacker's. "Seriously. Dimbulb . . . Dimitri . . . is bad news. I know that because I can't get the bastard off my back, even though I've made it very clear that I'm taken. This should be easy for you. He's a jerk. He doesn't even like you, let alone love you. Forget about him. Once you do, you'll have time for Mr. Right, whoever he *really* is."

Lenore stood silently for a moment. Then, quietly, she said, "I can't change the way I feel."

Mia just shook her head. "Yeah, but you can't change reality either, honey."

The only response Lenore could come up with was a sulk.

"Come on," Mia said cheerily, throwing an arm around Lenore's shoulders. "Let's forget this crap for now and get to class."

Lenore gave in and allowed Mia to march her toward the lecture hall door.

"Just think," Mia said. "If that homeless guy *had* wacked you, you would have missed the first day of summer session Human Sexuality. And *quel* tragedy *that* would have been!"

2

Feeling better due to her mercurial friend's ministrations, Lenore fell giggling with Mia through the lecture hall door. Below, other students were still milling on risers. The professor's desk, to the left at the lowest level of the hall, stood empty before a room-width chalkboard. Beside the desk sat several large cardboard boxes.

Between the age of the building and the heat emanating from students in waves, the room reeked of sweat, academia and apathy.

"Hey, Lenore, get into a fight?" asked a voice just behind Lenore. She and Mia turned to find a smug-faced Dimitri. Lenore's immediate blush of shame deepened to a rich shade of pride as she realized that he'd spoken to her first.

"Hey, Mia," Dimitri continued, instantly ignoring Lenore. "See this biceps?"

He raised one sculptured arm and flexed it, showing off a bulging biceps.

"It's toned cuz I've been imagining you on my arm for an hour every day!" His eyes threw grappling hooks of desire toward Mia.

They fell well short.

Mia just sneered and held up her middle finger. "Imagine yourself on *this* for an hour every day, Dimbulb!"

"Try me," he replied without hesitation.

"Eeeww!!" Mia said and pulled Lenore away from Dimitri. "Come on. Zander saved us some seats. Oh, crap. He's with his stoner buddy Aiden."

Lenore had one last glimpse of Dimitri before Mia tugged her to the opposite side of the lecture hall.

Dimitri appeared to stare after them, his self-confident expression plastered on his face. But Lenore knew the truth: his eyes only saw Mia.

"Stop that!" Mia said as she pushed Lenore roughly down into a seat. "Lenny, baby, really," Mia said, plopping herself into the chair between Lenore and Zander. "The guy's a self-centered pig. The only reason he's after me, or any girl, is that he knows he'll never physically be able to fuck himself."

"Don't be gross."

"Aversion training, honey. I'm trying to help you break the habit."

"Hey guys," said Zander. Long, brown bangs covered half his face. Mia reached instinctively to brush them away.

"Hey tiger." Practically leaping into his chair, she kissed him. Copiously.

On the other side of Zander, his friend Aiden waved at Lenore, a dopey grin plastered to his face. Lenore smiled back, but she didn't feel like having a conversation over two chairs filled with hot classroom love, so she turned back to sneak another look at Dimitri. He continued to stare in their direction. His smug expression melted as he watched Mia with Zander. Anger took its place.

Without disengaging from Zander, Mia pinched Lenore.

"How's my baby?" Mia asked Zander when she finally came up for air.

"Your baby's fine," he said, breathing heavily, Mia clinging to him like a muffler. "How 'bout you, Lenore? How's it going?"

"Oh, it goes," Lenore shrugged noncommittally.

"It doesn't just *go,* honey," Mia said. "Tell him what happened outside just now."

Zander gave her his polite attention, but Lenore just shrugged.

"It was nothing."

"Nothing, my ass!" As usual, Mia took it upon herself to deliver news like a breathless reporter during an attack by Godzilla. "Lenny was attacked by a homeless man outside the building. He almost killed her!"

"Oh, please!" Lenore said, rolling her eyes. "He was scared or something. He was looking for a friend."

"Wow!" Aiden blurted out. He had a habit of interjecting dramatic non sequiturs into other people's conversations. He did not disappoint. "You should hear what happened to me last night."

"You get attacked, too?" Mia asked.

"Naw. But check *this* out," he continued. "Me and my roommate saw UFOs last night."

"Like, as in flying saucer?" Mia asked.

"Oh, come on," Lenore said.

"Seriously. There were these big orange lights. They just zoomed around the campus, split up and disappeared."

Lenore and Mia exchanged a skeptical look.

"When did this happen, sweetie?" Mia asked.

"Like, on our way home from the bars, and—"

"Coming home from the bars and you saw something strange? Well, I never!" Mia always applied sarcasm liberally to the affected area. Her tone, however, was lost on Aiden. "I bet we'll find out about cattle mutilations and the abductions soon."

Mia seemed ready to let loose another acid-coated comment when the professor shuffled in from a lower-level door. He entered as if in deep thought, looking to the ground and absently stroking his ponytail.

The dull roar of pre-class conversation subsided immediately. The professor sat heavily on the corner of the desk at the front of the hall. Folds of flesh from his thighs oozed over the edges of the desk. The class quieted completely by the time he finished surveying the room with bright, heavy-lidded eyes.

"All right, people," he began. Though his features said India, his accent said Harvard. His voice filled the lecture hall without electronic amplification. "My name is Professor Ajit Waman. This class is Human Sexuality 101. It's the first day of the second summer session." Then, without changing his almost monotone delivery, he asked, "Are we having fun yet?"

No one laughed. By the look on Waman's face, no amusement had been intended.

The professor's heavy-lidded eyes scanned the room as he continued to sit on the corner of the desk, his hands thrust into his pockets and one leg swinging absently.

Suddenly, as if in response to a question only he heard, he shook his head with fatherly disappointment, his ponytail whipping from side to side. Professor Waman hefted himself off the desk with his hands, and once standing, stuffed them back into his pockets before starting to pace. His gaze dropped to the floor again, and he addressed the class almost as if he were talking to himself. Even so, his voice never failed to reach the back row.

"I know how it is with you kids. Reading's not your thing. It's all video games and sports and local television news. So in addition to the reading we'll be doing this session—and we *will* be reading, people—today we'll begin a little ongoing experiment, something I'm sure you'll all find 'interactive.' "

Without taking his hands from his pockets, he nodded at one of the students in the front row.

"You. See those boxes behind my desk? Open one up," he commanded. The student in the front row, an acne-riddled freshman, froze like a deer in headlights. The professor just stood in front of the student and stared, embarrassing the boy into standing up and walking to the boxes.

"You might think that in this class you will learn the right way to please your woman. Or man."

This elicited several snickers, but again, Professor Waman's flat delivery and grave expression indicated he was not delivering a stand-up routine.

"You'll certainly learn where the basic plumbing is, though if you don't know it at this point, I pity you. No, you people are going to learn the *real* lesson of Human Sexuality. It's called 'responsibility.'"

The students exchanged nervous glances. Mia pretended to jam her finger down her throat. No one liked where this was going.

The professor turned to the pimply student and waved his hand impatiently. "Take one out," he said, then turned back to the class. "People, meet a new addition to each of your families."

The student hesitated slightly and reached into the box. Lenore thought he was close to soiling his pants, if he had not done so already. When he held up what he'd retrieved from the box, several students gasped. It was a five-pound bag of flour.

A male voice from the back of the room groaned, "You've got to be kidding!"

Professor Waman's heavy eyes flicked briefly in that direction. A smile flashed on his lips and was gone so quickly that it might have been a hallucination of a smile.

A hand shot up among the students. "With all due respect, Professor Waman, isn't caring for bags of flour a high school assignment?"

This time, Waman did smile. "Yes. And no." Then he paused, as if a new and strange thought struck him. "This is a lecture hall, no? So I will lecture."

With that, he began his slow, eyes-down pacing.

"In high school, you had relatively little freedom. You lived with your parents, had curfews, your social experiences were relatively limited and your perspectives immature. You have probably changed more as people in your time since high school than you did in the previous eight years of your life. Many of you live alone, far from your parents. You have roommates, girl-friends and boyfriends—some of you couples even live together. Others of you might even be married already. Your freedom now is infinitely greater—no curfews, you can party openly rather than experience the vicarious thrills of fruit-flavored wine in the basement of your house while your parents are asleep. If you don't want to get out of bed and come to class, you are free to do so. The university already has your money, whether you attend any given class or not. Now, whether this

has made any of you more mature is another matter
entirely."

Professor Waman finally took his hands from his
pockets and began to rub them together. He watched
himself do this as he continued to talk.

"Okay people, this is how it will work. Each student
in this class will be paired with another. The pair will be
given a bag of flour to care for as if it were your own
child. The child must always be attended to by one or
the other parent—if the 'spouses' live in separate apartments, then a custody-sharing arrangement must be
made. But at no time can the child be left alone, unless
someone arranges for a baby-sitter. Otherwise, a child
must go with you wherever you go, the way it would be
if you had a child.

"Families will keep a log of all activities. Did you
just place the child in a corner and ignore him while
you and your friends watched television, or did you sit
him on your lap? How did you carry him or her in pub-
lic? Papoose-style? Did you push a stroller? I will pay
special attention to how parents solved conflicts where
the child and its care are concerned.

"You must above all provide for the safety and well-
being of your child, making certain he or she comes to
no harm. Any signs of abuse or neglect, such as tears or
punctures in the packaging, crumpled corners, or even
showing up to class without your child, will be grounds
for failing the assignment. And the class."

A wave of distress washed through the room.

"As to your behavior outside of this hall," Professor Waman continued, "remember, people, this is a college town. If you go bar-hopping with your friends and neglect your child, there's a good chance I'll find out about it, so take this very seriously. Very seriously, indeed."

The room went utterly silent as each student considered the assignment. And how many loopholes they could think of.

3

A t that moment, on the other side of the campus, a group of seven young men was noisily and agonizingly vocalizing in one of the Weaver Music Building's many rehearsal rooms. The offending singers went by the name of The Shower Tones. Anyone with the stomach to listen to them for more than a few seconds would have picked out the old barbershop chestnut "Coney Island Baby"—and found it wormy.

This lack of collective musical ability had earned the group the nickname of The Loser Tones across the campus. Their performances at the various dorm "coffeehouses," campus benefits, and sleepy off-campus bars had the humorous and dreadful inevitability of a giant zit on the tip of one's nose—they always drew a large, snickering crowd who used gargantuan effort not to point at the obvious and laugh out loud.

Music students rushed past the doorway when The Shower Tones were rehearsing, painfully aware of how much the group butchered the form.

"Wait, wait, wait!" Quincy Peterson shouted, his speaking voice considerably higher than his baritone singing. The other singers trailed off raggedly. "Can we narrow it down to only two or three tempos, if we can't manage a single one?"

The other Shower Tones gaped at him dumbly.

"I vote we sing it 'andale,' " chirped Flutie, the heavyset first tenor. "Besides, it'll be over faster. Right, Thomas?"

"That's 'andante,' you ignoramus," said one of the bass singers. "We gotta do this different, like slow and sexy. Like Luther."

Luther Vandross was Thomas Tinker's personal hero. Thomas always referred to his idol by his first name, always with a slight tremble in his voice. To hear him tell it, Luther not only possessed "God's voice" but was also an expert in social and political affairs, science and a master chef.

Trevin Joyner, one of the two second tenors, rolled his eyes and shook his head. He opened his mouth to speak, then stopped, as if the jostling erased his short-term memory. All eyes were on him. Closing his mouth, he took a deep breath, closed his eyes and seemed to say a prayer. Watching Trevin prepare to talk was like watching a dog walk in circles for minutes on end until it finally lay down.

"But . . . but . . . barbershop *isn't* slow and sexy, Thomas," Trevin finally said. Then he took another deep breath and turned to Flutie.

Ty, the other first tenor, countered, saying, "It's not a train without brakes, either."

Then everyone's voices swelled, arguing on how exactly the song should be handled. After several rebuffs, Quincy finally got them to quiet down again.

"We'll wait for Buddy to arrive," he said, stifling further debate. "He'll sew this all together."

"Buddy?" asked Uni, who had remained mostly silent during the debate.

He was the youngest of the group, a seventeen-year-old computer genius and Japanese exchange student. He also sang a surprisingly clear bass. He was also one of the newer members of the group and had not yet developed the appreciation for their absent leader that his cohorts had.

"Buddy idiot," he said, much more practiced with machine language than the English language. "We should no listen to Buddy."

The older members of the group practically choked on the younger boy's blasphemy. Wes, the energetic freshman with aspirations to a career in theme-park performance, spoke up in Uni's defense.

"He's right, guys," Wes said, putting a supportive hand on Uni's shoulder, who shrugged it off with an uncomfortable glare. "Buddy's my boy and all, you know what I'm saying, but if he's so great, why is he late? There's no 'I' in team, you know what I'm saying? And being late is very 'I.' "

Just then the doorknob jiggled and the door opened. Everyone turned to watch. As all had expected, and some had fervently hoped, in strode Nicholas "Buddy" Bragg. Considered by many to be the Clown Svengali of Oxford, he was several years older than the other students in the room. He was supposed to have graduated two years earlier, but his class schedule was light enough, and his underachievement consistent enough, that he seemed only to aspire to being a career student. With his academic career on autopilot, he devoted himself to cultivating sycophants among the incoming students, which he did based on his looks and charm. And his prospectives lack thereof. With his broad, easygoing smile, his ability to ease into any social situation, he seemed like the cool upperclassman that every naïve underclassman wanted to grow up and be one day. And if nothing else, maybe they could score with his cast-off chicks.

The door clicked shut behind Buddy. Using the sound as a cue, he stopped, deliberately posing in a casual stance. Sensing tension in the room, he picked out the division between the new freshman and the rest of the group. He'd have to deal with the problem quickly. He'd had a strange and wonderful dream the night before, one that required group harmony on several different levels. So, with Uni and Wes in his crosshairs, he set his smile to stun.

"Radical shorts, Wes," he said, joining the group. "Where do you get all that fine gear? Man oh man!"

"Wal-Mart," Wes said, blushing. "I just have an eye, you know, homeboy?"

"Uni," Buddy said. "Who's the man?" They shared an elaborate handshake Buddy had taught Uni. He knew it made the freshman feel like more than a brain-on-a-stick, which was how his parents and most other students viewed him.

Insinuating himself between Wes and Uni, he put his arms around both of them chummily. Both were instantly at ease.

"So what's the buzz, fuzz?" He dialed his smile down to the level of an ultra-suave tractor beam.

"It's 'Coney Island Baby,' " Quincy told him. "It's just not coming together."

"No worries," Buddy said. "Cuz I got some news for yous!"

The music he had dreamed about switched on in his head. Even though no one else in the room heard it, he bopped his head to the beat.

"I had a dream I wanna share with you," he said, his body joining the act as if he were in a funk-trance. With one hand he conducted an invisible orchestra; the other lightly patted the top of his gel-frozen dark hair. "We're changing up."

"W-w-what?" asked Trevin. "We've been rehears-ing."

"Like cats on a back fence at midnight," snorted Thomas. "No soul. No smoothness."

"In my dream, we found our souls and brought on the smoothness," Buddy told them.

The others regarded him with a mixture of awe and confusion. He flashed his smile again, then added a wink for extra reassurance.

"Check it out," Buddy said, the groove in his voice. "I didn't just have a dream, I had a *funky* dream last night." On the cue inside his head, his hips started gyrating. The groove overtook him entirely now. He was sweating funk.

"Yeah! A funky dream!" Buddy shimmied his shoulders up and down, snapping in rhythm.

"Oooo, too funky!" Buddy turned to one side, hip-swayed forward two steps, rocked in time to the other side and hip-swayed back.

"Uh, uh . . . uh, uh!" he grunted, performing a rhythmically perfect, yet almost inhumanly cramped, body contortion which appeared to bend his elbows, knees and ankles the wrong way. His head bobbed on his neck like an animated Egyptian hieroglyphic.

"And now the big finish," he announced. Taking one exaggerated step backwards, he launched himself into spin, knee bent and hands in the air, then leaped forward, landing on his knees and sliding forward. He came to an abrupt stop, tearing his shirt open. "Uh!!!"

The only sound in the room for several seconds was the clicking of buttons, which had torn off Buddy's shirt, as they bounced onto the floor.

"How hot was that?" It wasn't a question. It was a challenge.

"Uh, what *was* that, Buddy?" Quincy finally asked meekly.

"I dunno," said Thomas. "Looks like Buddy was getting down with his bad self there."

"You got it, Thomas," Buddy said. "And that was just the choreography."

"For what?" asked Ty.

"For our new *thing*." At the moment, the group was too shocked to get his meaning.

"Backstreet, *NSYNC, 98 Degrees . . ." The blank stares started to give way to panic. At least it was beginning to register. So he laid out his dream.

"We're gonna become a boy band, guys!"

4

The pairings assigned for the parenthood experiment added to the turmoil in the class. Geeks were matched with the pretty and the popular. Punker chicks found themselves "married" to jocks. In many couples, religious beliefs—or worse, diet preferences—clashed. The harmonized discord seemed meticulously planned by Professor Waman.

Perhaps the only well-matched couple in the room was a pair of infamous sophomores, Rosenberg and Gyllenhal. The two had been among the few survivors of the Tragedy of Cameron Dean, Captain of the Globe Monarchs, as it was known on campus. In that fateful trip to Denmark, many students had been slaughtered by what was still subject to rumor. Some reports told of an escaped mental patient running amok in a castle that Dean had inherited. Other voices, in much quieter tones, spoke of a vengeful ghost. This rumor had been started by the football player's roommate, Harry

Wilkins. But these had been some of Harry's last words. He now sat silent in a local psychiatric hospital, rocking back and forth in a chair, holding his sides.

Somehow, Ben Rosenberg and Pete Gyllenhal had emerged unscathed. And deeply in love. More importantly, they possessed the only photographic evidence of the event, pictures that became the focus of a bidding war by major news organizations and book publishers. This was their first semester back. They had returned to school very rich young men.

They were also the only two members of the class actually looking forward to the assignment. At the other end of the spectrum was Mia, who dragged Aiden, her husband by assignment, and Zander to the front of the class. She confronted Professor Waman with a great heave of her shoulders and an indignant pair of crossed arms.

"I want a divorce," she huffed. *"Before* we have kids. My real boyfriend is in this class." She shoved Zander forward as if presenting a slave for auction. "So let me just swap him for Aiden."

Aiden tilted his head and shrugged. "That's cool with me, Professor."

"Spouse swapping, Ms. Miller? Hardly a healthy family dynamic for an infant, wouldn't you say?" Without raising his voice, it seemed to fill the lecture hall more powerfully than before.

Not to be denied, Mia channeled her indignation into a pathetic whine.

"But he's a *drug* user!" She pointed to Aiden, who again shrugged.

"Is it 4:20 yet?" he giggled. No skin off his nose.

"See?" said Mia. "That's bad for children."

"Well, then he will be judged on how that affects his performance of the assignment, don't you think?" Waman remained utterly unruffled. "And as for you, having to live with no guarantee of getting your way all the time will prove to be your true challenge. Please go before I grade you here and now."

Mia gasped. Loudly. "How dare you?!" she hissed. Still, the professor remained implacable.

"I don't *dare*, Ms. Miller," he said. "I *assign*. As for you"—he turned to the class, which had fallen cemetery silent—"as for all of you, you pass. Or you fail."

Zander tugged on Mia's arm. "Come on, honey. Aiden, grab your kid."

Zander dragged Mia huffing and puffing back to her seat.

"Let's call him Stoney," Aiden giggled as he caught up with them, holding a bag of flour.

Zander convinced Aiden to care for the "baby Stoney" that night so Mia could calm down. But Zander's assignment as Lenore's husband only agitated her further.

Lenore tried to act enthusiastic when Zander became her husband. Truly, things could have been worse. But deep down, she had hoped the professor would have paired her with Dimitri. Instead, a thin, pallid girl named Ione Delacorte became his wife. She had large eyes and spoke mostly in questions, as if the universe were quickly unfolding its wonders to a mind that tried in vain to press a cosmic Pause button. Lenore knew that this pleasant, vacuous quality would suit Dimitri just fine. Besides, he would easily convince Ione to care for their "child."

Like his own father, Dimitri was not fond of children. Had Dimitri not learned how to play poker at an early age, his father wouldn't have paid him any attention at all. As for Ione, if she didn't mind him being an absent father, class would be a cakewalk for him.

"Can you believe that guy?" Mia demanded to know after class.

"Relax, baby," Zander told her. "It's just homework."

"Yeah, but—"

"Hey, Mia," Dimitri said, suddenly stepping in front of the group.

"What do you want, Dimbulb?"

"Pet names mean you love me," Dimitri responded with a fake swoon. "So my wife's got the kid tonight. Looks like *your* hubby's playing Mr. Mom. So how about dinner tonight?"

"Puh. Leaze." Mia replied. "Like I'm going to have dinner with you."

"Um, Dimitri, I'm standing right here," Zander said.

"Yeah? And?" Dimitri barely looked away from Mia. "Okay. We'll figure out something. Meanwhile, tell your hubby to sing your baby to sleep," he said. "That's what my housekeeper used to do for me. She said it kept the monsters away."

Too soon for Lenore, not soon enough for Mia, he walked away.

"More like the monsters were afraid of *him*," said Mia. "What a freak. Is it me, or is he getting all stalky?"

"Leave him alone, you guys," Lenore began before she could stop herself.

Zander and Mia rolled their eyes in unison. Zander spoke up first.

"I forgot," he said mildly. "You have a crush on him. Speaking of unexplainable phenomena, anyone want to come UFO hunting with me tonight?"

"UFO hunting? Sweetie, you've got to be kidding."

"I'm not. I believe Aiden. They may come back. I wanna check that out."

Lenore held up the bag of flour she carried.

"Well, I'm betting UFO watching will be after baby's bedtime. So we can't both go."

"I'm sorry," Zander said. "I almost forgot. You want me to take it tonight? What is *it*, anyway? A boy or a girl?"

Neither had given the matter much thought. All three examined the bag for any sign that would help them "sex" their child. For good or for ill, the bags of flour were not anatomically detailed. Finally, Lenore and Zander agreed that they shared a son named Rolf.

Lenore volunteered to care for Rolf that night, leaving Zander free to search for UFOs.

"Really wish you could come with us," Zander told her.

"It'd be fun," Lenore said. "But might as well take this assignment seriously."

"Puh. Leaze." Mia regarded them both as if they were insane. "You with the UFOs, like they exist in the first place and even if they did, why would they come here? Then *you* with the flour baby. Like Waman's gonna see you if you put the stupid bag of flour on the counter and leave the house. I swear, you guys."

"If you don't wanna come out tonight, Mia, then why don't you baby-sit for Lenore and the two of *us* will hunt for UFOs?"

"Oh, right," said Mia. "Like I'm gonna leave the two of you alone. Don't want Lenore developing a crush on you like she has on Dimbulb."

"Mia!" Both Lenore and Zander spoke at the same time.

"Nah, that's okay," Lenore said quickly. "I wanna stay in tonight anyway."

"I'm only joking, sweeties!" Mia said. "Puh. Leaze." Then she hugged Zander close. "You couldn't take my sweet thang away from me if you tried. Guess I gotta thank Dimbulb for something, cuz I know how delicious my little Zander is."

Zander started to blush from the attention, and Mia noticed.

"Look at that! Cute or what?" She finally released him. "Anyway, where my boy goes, so do I. Even if it's to fight the aliens."

"We don't know that they're hostile," Zander pointed out.

"They always are, honey, they always are. How could something from another world land here, take a look around and *not* get pissed at us?"

5

Later that night, Zander spent two uneventful hours with Mia wandering through the Globe campus, looking for strange lights in the sky. It was a half an hour until midnight. The sun had gone down hours ago, and the mercury never threatened to sink. Climbing halfway up the football field bleachers, Zander finally sat down. Mia plopped beside him, too tired and sticky for the cuddling she had intended to initiate. He leaned back on his elbows against the bleachers and gazed skyward.

Irritated by his inattention, Mia grabbed his nose and pulled his face toward hers.

"Owww!" he cried nasally and pulled away.

"Give it a rest, Zander," she told him. "Look at me for once instead of the stupid sky!"

Zander massaged his nose. "But I don't wanna miss the UFOs if they come back!" He returned to his search. Mia went for his nose again, but he anticipated her attack and scooted away across the aluminum bench.

"You think they'd be here two nights in a row?" she said. "If you were an alien from another planet, would *you* stick around in Stratford?"

"I guess you're right."

"Puh. Leaze. Of course I'm right." Mia lowered her voice to a sexy growl. "I only came out here cuz I thought we could mess around. There are a few places on campus we haven't done it yet."

Zander snickered and brought his face back toward hers.

"I forgot about that."

"How could you forget?" Mia was practically purring. Their noses touched. "Now kiss me and let's go somewhere where's there's air-conditioning."

"Yeah?"

"Yeah. And then let's see if we can break it."

"Mmmmmm . . . ," he responded, leaning forward to kiss her as they straddled the bench.

The heat, the humidity and the hunt for aliens were momentarily forgotten. Mia gently but firmly forced him backwards, nearly causing him to lose his balance. Finally he succumbed to the inevitable and lay back against the cool aluminum bench. As he settled into place, Mia climbed on top of him, having accomplished the entire maneuver without once withdrawing her tongue from his mouth.

Quite masterfully, they performed quite a variety of wet-sounding acts upon each other without a single loss of balance. Twenty minutes later, Zander finally found

Mia beneath him. For several minutes after that, they simply stared into each other's eyes. The night had fallen silent and comfortable around them, as if it had covered them with a blanket.

"So I figure it's time we got married, Zander," Mia said suddenly.

"Huh?" He immediately pulled back to get a better view of her face, to see if she were maybe joking. Or insane.

"Well, we've been going together for about a year now, it's pretty serious and—puh leaze—like either of us will find anyone more perfect for each other!" The words rushed out, as if she were a squirrel chattering at Zander from a tree. "You can move into my family's house—get out of that icky apartment of yours—until I buy a house of our own. I'll be a lawyer, probably, at least that's what's supposed to happen, and you can get a new band together—with you as lead singer, I mean, Kev's nice but he's got no *it*, ya know?—and I'll support you while you pursue your music career. How perfect is that?"

"But—" Zander's eyes were beginning to glaze over.

"I know," Mia said, not noticing Zander's rising panic. "It's very Sadie Hawkins of me. Do you even know what that means? It's where the girl asks the boy to a dance. That's how my mom snagged my dad, by asking him to a Sadie Hawkins dance years ago. Come to think of it, I think they met at the dance and ditched their dates, but they met at a Sadie Hawkins dance. The point being that you don't have to feel less of a man for me asking and not you. I mean, these are the Oughts. And we *ought* to be able to do what we want by now, and I *want* to marry you."

The night fell silent again as Zander struggled for the air that Mia had consumed with her daisycutter marriage proposal.

"By the way," she added quickly, just as he opened his mouth to respond, "I'll probably wanna hyphenate my last name, so I won't lose my identity completely, but I'm sure you won't mind that, right, sweetie?"

Zander snapped his mouth shut.

"Holy shit!" Mia suddenly cried, sitting up quickly and knocking Zander off the bench.

From his back, wedged between the risers, Zander could see what Mia saw: two glowing orange balls of light. Mia pulled him back up onto the bench just as the lights disappeared over the edge of the stadium, heading across campus.

The acrid, sweet smell hit Aiden the moment he opened the door to the apartment he shared with fellow stoner Carter Chirocco.

"Dude, what's burning?" Aiden asked.

"Oh, dude! Whoa!" Carter hopped up from the sidewalk-rescue sofa and disappeared into the kitchen. Sublime blared from the speakers, and *Dude Where's My Car?* flashed on the TV screen.

Aiden set down his guitar and tumbled over the back of the couch to a sitting position. Practice with his rock band, The Sizzle Zits, had not gone that well that night. The lead singer just had not been mellow, so rehearsal had broken up early. Putting his feet up on the coffee table, he nearly kicked over a bong filled with mouthwash.

"Dude!" he called out. "Like could it be, like, any hotter in here? Seriously!"

His roommate's only response was to bang the oven shut. Aiden figured he couldn't hear over the music and the movie, both of which were playing at full volume. At least the burning smell was dissipating. Whatever it was, it must have only just started burning when Aiden returned home. He shook his head.

"Dude! You're gonna burn this place down one day, ya brainless git!" He waited a moment for a response, and then became distracted by the image on the television of a dog smoking a pipe. "This movie busts me up!"

"Voilà, dude!" Carter called from the doorway to the kitchen. In his hands he held a plate stacked high with brownies.

"Awesome!"

Carter set the plate down on the coffee table, also nearly knocking over the bong. Aiden grabbed a brownie and stuffed it into his mouth.

"I tried to scrape off the burned parts," Carter said through his own mouthful of brownie.

"Sweet!" Aiden mumbled, crumbs dropping into his lap. Though a faint charred taste remained, the brownies were pretty rad. After taking another big bite, Aiden examined the brownie. As he expected, it contained many small, green leafy bits. "Sweet!" he mumbled again.

"Yeah, dude. Got the munchies."

"This is only gonna give us more munchies, dude," Aiden pointed out. "If we keep eating them, we'll never NOT have the munchies. It's a vicious cycle."

Both giggled like schoolgirls at the notion of perpetually consuming pot brownies. By the time they polished off the entire plate, the movie was just ending and the words "bow wow wow yippee yo yippee yay" coming from the stereo speakers proclaimed that Snoop Doggy Dogg was in the hizzouse. Or at least on the CD changer.

Aiden floated up from the couch.

"Want a beer, dude?" It came out as one word: *wannabeerdude.*

"Nah dude, I wanna beer *chick.*" Carter sculpted an impossibly proportioned figure of a woman in the air with his hands. "Like a Hooters girl. And hell, she doesn't even have to be that classy!"

"Don't be a smart-ass," Aiden told him and went for a couple of long, tall ones.

The mess in the kitchen stopped him in his tracks. White or brown powder covered every countertop. Chocolate chips littered the powder-covered floor like rat turds on a Côte d'Azur beach. In the sink, a batter-laden spatula protruded from a sludgy glass mixing bowl. Aiden immediately thought of Excalibur—one that only the Pillsbury Doughboy could wield. The only comfort he drew from the bakery carnage was the absence of green flecks.

At least Carter hadn't wasted the *important* ingredients.

From the kitchen doorway, he turned back to Carter.

"What's this shit, Martha Stewart?" he asked. "You can't use a mix like the rest of us?"

"These kind of brownies have to be from scratch, dude," Carter replied, as if that explained everything.

Aiden snorted at him. It came louder than he had intended, so as he returned to the kitchen, he continued snorting, experimenting with different volumes and pitches to find just the right snorting sound. Pulling out two bottles of beer from the fridge, he saw the bag of flour.

The bottles nearly slipped from his hands.

"Stoney!" The bag was nearly empty.

From the living room, Carter called out, "Dude, where's my beer? Where's my beer, dude? Dude, where's my beer?"

This time, the bottle in Aiden's right hand did slip out as a fit of giggles washed over him. Luckily, his hand was over the counter and he was able to set the bottle down, a little too hard. Beer foamed out of the bottle and streamed down the sides. It mixed with the flour and sugar on the counter, immediately forming a paste.

"What's up, Aiden, man?" Carter called out again.

Aiden lost control of his laughter. He quickly put down the second bottle of beer and leaned against the counter. Rocking forward and back, he almost hit his forehead against the counter.

"You baked Stoney, man!" Aiden's body contracted in a fresh burst of hysterical laughter.

This time, instead of Carter's voice, a crash sounded from the living room. In his condition, Aiden barely noticed, briefly thinking that the bong had finally met its maker. Behind him, he heard Carter step into the kitchen and stop at the doorway.

As he turned toward his roommate, Aiden doubled over in laughter once more. Tears streamed from his eyes. He gasped, unable to catch his breath.

"Dude, dude," he said, trying to wipe the tears away. He couldn't see. "We ate my baby!"

That was too much for him. Aiden sank to his knees, into the sugar, cocoa powder, chocolate chips and flour. It was all he could do to keep himself from falling to the floor in a fetal position and rolling around in hysterics.

Then he noticed that Carter wasn't laughing. And that he hadn't moved from the doorway.

Aiden rubbed his eyes again, clearing his vision. Still on his knees, he was wracked by another spasm of giggles and forced it back. Carter began to move toward him silently.

But it wasn't Carter.

The first things he saw were the intruder's feet. But they weren't feet, per se. Certainly not human ones.

They were hooves. Cloven hooves. Like the devil's.

Aiden jerked his gaze upward, quickly taking in the powerful, furry legs, claws at the end of equally muscular arms, broad shoulders. Like a football player or a bouncer, the thing's head sat directly upon its shoulders. A cowl of black fur framed a fang-filled mouth, silently snarling and smiling at the same time. The nose was the snout of a beast, the eyes intelligent and glowing with deadly intent. Upon its brow were set two gnarled horns.

Aiden's laughter died instantly.

He watched as it strode slowly and heavily toward him. It looked down at him, breathing, its expression a beacon of malevolent delight.

Laughter consumed Aiden again, and he fell howling onto his side. He rolled in place, his body coating itself in brownie ingredients. He held his sides, as if he would soon burst from laughter. His eyes squeezed shut again, tears and powder mixing to create trails of brownie batter on his face.

The precise moment when Aiden's laughter became screams of terror was hard to tell. But the apartment fell completely silent soon thereafter.

6

The trucks appeared at three-thirty in the morning, approaching from the west. There were two of them, well-traveled eighteen-wheelers, one a half-mile behind the other, headlights stabbing through thick, hazy air. A caravan of ragtag vehicles followed the trucks down the two-lane highway: a tour bus with a crooked, faded Happy Trails sign in the destination window; a few flatbed trucks sporting irregular bulges covered by oily tarps; several cars neutered of make or model by rust and primer.

About six miles outside of Stratford, the lead truck let out a horn blast and started to slow. Within a mile, it had stopped completely. Its cab was dark, and only vague shapes could be seen within, had there been anyone around to observe. The highway was utterly deserted, save for the strange caravan. The truck's engine idled roughly, as if it, not the driver, was considering what to do next. The vehicles behind it all paused similarly.

Suddenly, the lead truck let out another blast from its horn and the engine roared back to life. A dozen other revving engines seemed to answer it. The truck pulled forward, then turned onto a dirt road that quickly disappeared into an empty field of scorched grass. The rest of the vehicles followed. Turning to face the town once more, the lead truck stopped again with a hydraulic whine. The second truck turned and pulled parallel to the first. The bus did the same, followed in turn by the rest of the caravan. Soon, all the vehicles sat in a line, all facing Stratford, their headlights appearing as solid cones in the humid air. The engines idled for nearly a minute, as if the vehicles were an armada preparing to invade the town.

Then, all at once, the engines cut out. Every pair of headlights died at the same time.

The doors of the bus folded open with a hiss of air, and dark figures marched out from both entrances. Similar shadows emerged from the trucks. Cargo doors for each eighteen-wheeler were rolled up, and tarps were pulled from the flatbeds.

And without a word, without light, the strange new arrivals went to work.

7

Mia nearly tackled Lenore as they arrived at Professor Waman's class the next morning. Mia was bursting at the seams.

"What?" Lenore asked. Setting Rolf on the desk in front of her, Lenore noticed that the desk on the other side of Mia was empty. "Where's Zander?"

"Running late, and it's driving me up a wall! Where have you been? I tried you like a zillion times last night!"

Mia clutched the arms of her chair and hopped up and down as she talked. Lenore had never seen her friend like this.

"Yeah," she said slowly. "I saw your number on my caller ID this morning."

Someone pushed past Lenore and Mia, flinging his backpack upon the desk. Zander poured himself into his seat. If he had showered, his bedraggled appearance hid it well. Mia reached over and stroked his arm.

"You look terrible, sweetie. Didn't sleep?"

"Hmmm . . . ," he replied groggily, rubbing his forehead.

"Me too! Too excited!" She turned back to Lenore. "Why didn't you answer your phone last night? You just won't believe the night we had last night!"

"I had the ringer off. It was late. I didn't want to wake the baby."

"Forget the frickin' baby, sweetie!" Mia nearly shouted, causing several nearby students to turn. "Zander and I saw the UFOs last night!"

"What?!" Lenore looked over to Zander, who was resting his chin on one hand, looking pale. He nodded almost imperceptibly.

"We were in the football stadium and they zoomed right over! Two big balls of light, just like that bonehead. I've never seen anything like it!" Suddenly, she turned on Zander. "Why didn't we bring a camera?! My dad's DV camera can catch things in low light. What were we thinking?"

"That they didn't exist," Zander mumbled.

Mia scowled and turned away from him.

"Were they flying saucers?" Lenore asked.

"No, more like balls of energy," Mia said. Again, Zander nodded in unenthusiastic agreement. "And not that big, but they sure weren't anything we've ever seen."

Despite the incredible news, Lenore could tell that Mia had more to say.

"And . . .?" she said.

"And that's not even the exciting part!" Mia's voice rose again.

"You didn't go on board or anything, did you?"

"No, silly!" Mia squeezed Zander close, as if for a photograph. "We're engaged! Could you die?!"

By the expression on Zander's face, he could.

"That's amazing!" Lenore said, her eyes immediately dropping to Mia's hand.

"Oh, there's no ring," Mia answered, wiggling her bare fingers. "I proposed. I figure we'll get a ring in a few weeks, whenever. No rush. We just decided, that's all. Isn't that awesome!"

"Yes, it is. I'm so happy for you both!"

They group-hugged. And Lenore was thrilled and jealous. And somewhere, way back there, hopeful.

"Maybe this will get Dimbulb off my back," Mia said, echoing Lenore's dim, hopeful thought.

Professor Waman entered the room a minute later. He approached the podium at an amble, unhurried, yet purposeful. The class quieted down long before he got to it. As before, he started class by standing there, hands in his pockets, surveying the room, blinking slowly.

"Welcome to day two of our little experiment," he droned. "I trust you all took great pains to make your children safe and comfortable."

He fell silent again. Many students shifted uncomfortably in their seats, unsure whether they were supposed to answer spontaneously or wait to be called upon. Professor Waman seemed to enjoy their discomfort, the ghost smile playing on his lips before disappearing once more.

"Pass your journals forward," he commanded.

The room filled with the sound of shuffling papers, like a strong wind in a forest.

"Shit!" Mia whispered. "I forgot to check with Aiden this morning." She quickly scanned the room. No Aiden. "Where the hell is he? I get the feeling Waman isn't going to take even a combined alien sighting and an engagement as an excuse for no homework."

Down at the front of the class, papers began to reach the first row. Waman directed Perry, the pimply freshman from the day before, to collect them while he went to his desk and withdrew an object from one of the lower drawers. Returning to the podium, he placed the object, a bag of flour, upon it.

"We'll hear some presentations in a moment." Then his eyes turned upward, focusing on a specific student. "First, Ms., ah, Miller. Yes. I understand you have no journal to hand in. Please come down to the podium."

"But Professor Waman, um . . ." Mia stood awkwardly.

"Fear not, Ms. Miller. You're in no trouble." The professor offered a benevolent smile. Mia pushed her way out of her row and approached tentatively.

"Aiden took our, um, child home last night, um, we didn't get to—"

Professor Waman raised a hand, silencing her.

"Mr. Freeman has dropped the class," Professor Waman announced. "Apparently, raising a child wasn't his . . . bag. Sadly, you have become a single mother."

He lifted the bag of flour from the podium and handed it to Mia. She accepted it automatically, too nervous to register what it was.

"What's this?" she asked, seeing that the bag was beige instead of white, like those previously handed out.

"Wheat flour, Ms. Miller," Professor Waman told her. "It occurred to me that our children lacked the diversity of our parents. And so, you're not only a single mother, you're a single Caucasian mother of a child of color."

Mia looked from the bag of wheat flour in her hands to the professor, dumbstruck.

"I look forward to your notes on your experience, Ms. Miller."

Professor Waman shooed Mia away from the podium, and she staggered back to her seat. She said only one thing and then fell silent for the rest of the class:

"Is that guy a wack-job, or is it just me?"

Professor Waman randomly called upon students to recount their previous evening's activities, to explain and, in some cases, defend decisions made regarding care of the faux children. He then pressed them to relate these experiences to ones they might actually have had.

Lenore perked up when Dimitri's name was called. He stood with his "wife," Ione.

"I keep a very clean house," Ione said in an airy voice. "My parents did, too, so I wouldn't be exposed to germs. I want to do the same for my child."

"You realize, of course, that some germs are *good* for children," the professor said to her. "A child not exposed to a germ develops no immunity to it. Do you want to raise a bubble boy, Ms. Delacorte? A child without the means to protect itself from the world and its contagions?"

Ione looked at him, befuddled and frowning. "No, Professor. But if I can protect my child the way my parents protected me, I want to do that. If I can give my baby a clean, disinfected floor to crawl on so he's safe, I think that's a good thing."

Waman regarded her for a moment, then nodded. "And you?" he said to Dimitri, who stood beside Ione, looking bored.

"Well, Professor, I don't know what to tell you. This isn't the family I'd have. The way I'd raise a child. I don't even love her."

"Humor me, Mr. Carlton. For the sake of this class." More ominously, he added, "For the sake of your grade."

"Well, humor *me* for a moment, Professor."

The class registered this apparent challenge. Waman and Dimitri stared at each other for a moment. Ione, cradling her bag of flour in her arms, seemed oblivious to the whole exchange. The professor's expression remained unreadable.

"Go on," he said.

"Isn't this a setup to fail, the way things go in real life?" Dimitri asked. "Like an arranged marriage, like marrying someone because of status or because it'll make your parents happy, because you irrationally just think you should? I mean, how am I supposed to raise a healthy child in a falsely constructed scenario?"

Waman nodded again but said nothing. Dimitri pointed toward Rosenberg and Gyllenhal. They sat side by side, a stroller folded flat between them, their "baby" held against Rosenberg's chest in a harness. Beside Gyllenhal's backpack sat a baby bag filled with bottles, formula, diapers, and more childcare accessories.

"Look at them," Dimitri said. "Would their baby be better off with those two gay guys together, or with one of them married to a woman, without her knowing that he's gay? If they had listened to what they 'should' do, then that's what would happen. A falsely constructed scenario. Bad for a kid."

"Fair enough," Waman told him. "So what are you saying?"

"I'm saying that I love someone else," Dimitri said, turning toward Mia.

"Great," Mia whispered. "Like I need this."

"For the sake of our child," he stated dramatically, pointing toward Mia, "as well as *her* child, I would rather be married to her, than take part in a sham marriage."

"And I thought Rosenberg and Gyllenhal were taking this assignment too seriously," Lenore whispered to Mia.

Waman looked from Mia to Dimitri.

"You make some good points, Mr. Carlton," Waman told him. "Though your motives are highly suspect. Still, sometimes, even in the best of circumstances, one finds oneself falling out of love, married to someone they realize it was a mistake to marry. Or conversely, they simply find someone else who is a greater inspiration for their love and passion. Do you simply turn your back on a spouse no longer desired, and the family you produced with her? Or do you work on it?"

Now Dimitri paused to think.

"Whatever the case, Professor, I think honesty is important."

"Granted. But if you're looking for a Mexican divorce here, you're not going to get it, Mr. Carlton. You'll remain in your pairing with Ms. Delacorte, and I will look forward to more of your observations on how to deal with a family situation that isn't entirely . . . ideal."

"But Mr. Waman—"

The professor waved his hand again, ending the conversation.

"Make it work, Mr. Carlton," he said. "Or choose to fail this class."

He motioned for Dimitri and Ione to sit down and turned to hear from a new couple.

8

The Old Man had gotten his nickname so long ago that even *he* thought of himself by that name. His wife, Mae, a quietly embattled woman, had been the first to call him Old Man. The great old farmhouse they used to share still seemed to creak with her footsteps, even though she had passed on many years ago. Nowadays, the Old Man lived alone within it, like a hermit inside the desiccated, hollowed-out corpse of a great dead whale.

Sometimes he got lonely. On days like today, he found the outside world too close for comfort.

"You don't like this one bit, do ya, Old Man?" he mumbled to himself, lowering the binoculars from his eyes.

Across his property, at the edge of the fields he let lie fallow this year, ran the barbed wire fence that separated his farm from the state-owned land. Normally that land beyond the fence was deserted. It certainly had been before bed last night. This morning, he found the horizon interrupted by trucks and tents and mechanical contraptions that had sprung up like a giant's weeds overnight.

He gave barely a thought as to how all that had been put together, right under his snoring old nose, so quickly, without waking him. Or why not a soul had stirred since he'd put the binoculars to his eyes and monitored the site beginning early this morning. He was more struck by what the appearance of a brightly colored proscenium, angry-looking wooden horses and a ramshackle Ferris wheel portended.

A carnival.

No, sir, the Old Man didn't like this one bit. It was practically on top of him, butted up against his property that way. The state should have informed him a carnival would camp there. But given its ragged gypsy look, like the traveling carnivals from his youth, he doubted the owners had even applied for anything as formal as a permit. He would have protested, in any event, having such a thing so close to his property, to his home. The carnival folk themselves were bad enough. Worse would be the crowds the infernal thing would attract. It'd only take one night for his own property to become a repository for empty beer bottles and used condoms.

Sitting there, the various unsafe-looking amusement rides and dirty tents rising from the plain looked like an elaborate mousetrap. A lot of work to put up, too. No doubt it'd take a lot of work to break it down.

But break it down they would, if the Old Man had anything to say about it. And the Old Man was never at a loss for words.

So he poked a finger in his old rotary phone and dialed. The scraping and whirring of the dial echoed through his house. Putting the phone to his ear, he waited for the distant ringing the ancient phone lines produced. Nothing.

The Old Man frowned, more out of irritation than surprise. He held the receiver button down with a spidery finger for a few seconds, then let go. Not even a click was heard from the line.

He replaced the phone in its cradle with a sigh. Living so far from town, his phone service had never been upgraded. There would be no broadband for him; he still got his television reception the old-fashioned way—with an aerial antenna. A computer had never been considered.

D-S-L my A-S-S, the Old Man thought to himself.

"Well, Old Man," he said out loud. "Looks like you're gonna have to have a talk with them carnies on your own. Call the sheriff later."

The Old Man was seventy, but he still stood over six feet tall and his eyes had lost little of the power that had won over a young Mae Archibald. The same set of eyes had stared down the government when it had threatened to take his land from him. A not-yet-Old-Man had grabbed his crotch and said to the government boy, "I got yer Eminent Domain right here."

He'd sent all the government boys packing. Carnies would be small fry.

On his way to his battered old Olds, the Old Man didn't even glance at the shotgun that stood propped up in a copper bucket near the front door, next to a tattered umbrella. He wasn't afraid of these carnie folk any more than he was afraid of getting himself a little wet.

The Olds choked to an oil-burning start, and he drove along the dirt road—dusty ruts carved in a field of scorched grass, really—toward the carnival. Dust billowed out behind the car like the train of a wedding gown. The windows were rolled up, and the vent pumped hot air. The car's AC had busted years ago. But that suited the Old Man just fine. He didn't notice the heat any more than he noticed cold or rain.

Only this carnival stuck in his craw. It wouldn't be lodged there for long, if he had his way. And he usually did.

At the edge of his property, the Old Man left the car and hopped the fence. His shirt cuff snagged on the barbed wire, but he pulled it free with one strong tug.

The carnival was deserted. Ghost town deserted. On the arch above the entrance, the words The Perpetuals' Fun Faire were painted in old English lettering. The canvas was worn, the paint cracked and pitted. It almost seemed as if the carnival had been here all along, rotting for summer after summer, and had only just appeared, like a Brigadoon of the Dead.

"Hello?!" he called out. The flapping of canvas in a hot summer breeze answered him.

The Old Man remembered seeing the peaks of tents on the opposite side of the carnival. While he could go around the perimeter, he decided simply to walk straight through the site. The walk would be shorter. Besides, if they felt comfy enough to appear uninvited, he felt no compunctions to entering uninvited himself.

They can punch my ticket later, he thought to himself.

One step past the entrance arch, the Old Man stopped abruptly. The world felt entirely different, as if he had stepped through a portal to another dimension. A brief and extraordinarily rare moment of panic set in. He could see out of the entrance archway—the empty ticket booth, the scorched earth, the barbed-wire fence in front of his car, and in the distance, his farmhouse. But he had the overwhelming feeling that he was trapped, like the images through the archway were an illusion, a photograph meant to fool him. Spinning around, he nearly jumped back through the arch. Dust crunched underfoot. And everything returned to normal. He was back in the real world. If he wanted, he could return to his property, get back into his car, and just plain forget about the carnival.

And the Old Man wanted to do this very much. The police could deal with this invasion. When the phone started working again.

"Ya damn fool!" he muttered to himself suddenly. "When'd ya ever hide behind authority, when it's you that usually sends authority into hidin'?"

And so the Old Man marched right back through that arch. And yes, he felt the same sort of strange dislocation he had felt before. But he ignored it. It was like the time he'd been shot (the one and only time he had ventured far out of Stratford and walked the streets of New York City), but he had ignored the sensation long enough to do what had had to be done. In that case, he had compartmentalized his discomfort until he and Mae had gotten to a hospital. In this case, he'd turn these gypsies, or whatever they were, away from his property.

Ahead and to his right lay the main mechanisms of the mouse trap, the Tilt-a-Whirl, an ancient Ferris wheel that looked more like a medieval torture device than an "amusement ride," and at the center of the cluster of rides, the merry-go-round. Except this round didn't look so merry. Instead of heading straight for the back of the park, toward the tents, he examined the rides. Up close, the horses looked frightened rather than angry. These horses were running desperately from some horror that appeared to be nipping at their haunches. And they seemed to realize, in their terror, that they were caught in a loop and would never escape.

The Old Man had to tear himself away from the merry-go-round for fear of actually seeing the creature pursuing the horses.

"May I help you?"

The Old Man jumped a foot in the air, spinning toward the sound of a woman's voice behind him.

"What the?—"

"I'm sorry, sir, I didn't mean to frighten you."

Her appearance was curious. She was evidently in her forties. Though she wore a dark skirt and business attire, her bronze skin and deep wrinkles told him that she was an outsider person, perhaps a farmer's wife. She smiled broadly and wore large, mirrored sunglasses.

"You didn't frighten me," the Old Man snapped. "You surprised me. That's different."

"Yes, of course," the woman agreed blandly. Her smile seemed pasted to her face. "What can I do for you?"

"I'll tell you what you can do, Miz . . . ," he trailed off, but the woman did not fill in the gap with her name. "Well, I'm here to ask you to leave."

This didn't faze her one bit, though she did make a show of briefly, if insincerely, biting her lip with concern. "Have we encroached upon your property?"

"No, in truth you haven't," said the Old Man. "But you're butted right up against it, snug as Tupperware after the burp. And the crowds you bring in are gonna cause trouble for me. Can't help but do so, being so close. And you know how people are."

"Yes, I do." The woman seemed to think for a moment. To the Old Man, it seemed a pretend pause, as if she could only *look* like she was thinking. "You should come meet the owners of the Perpetuals' Fun Faire. I'm sure we can make some sort of arrangement."

The Old Man snorted. "I'm not here to make any sort of *arrangement*, young lady."

"Please," she said, her smile widening even further. She offered her arm, and instinctively he took it. They began to walk across the carnival grounds. With each step, dust puffed into the air in little clouds.

"Frankly, sir, the owners hope not to attract the kind of business that would cause you trouble."

The Midway, filled with impossible-to-win games, passed by on their right. In their path ahead stood a metal pushcart. The glass case that sat on the cart seemed to be crusted pink.

"I'm sure the owners will address your concerns, sir," the woman went on. She touched his arm, as if they had become great friends.

Bragg grunted with frustration. "Now see here, young lady. Did your bosses get *any* sort of permission for your little carnival?"

"Fun Faire, sir. With an *E*."

"I don't care if you spell 'fun' with two *N*s, your little to-do shouldn't be here!"

The woman stopped them before the pushcart. The Old Man could see an aluminum cylinder, about two feet in diameter, sunk in the cart. Wisps of pink webbing stuck to everything. A sweet smell hung about the cart.

"Can I make you some cotton candy?"

"I don't eat that stuff. Let's just get on to your bosses."

All at once, the Old Man found his outrage fading. Here he was, in a place that reminded him of his youth, surrounded by the sweet smell of cotton candy, and in the company of a (*forgive-me-Mae*) attractive woman.

"It would be a mistake," she said, stepping behind the cotton candy machine, "for you to pass up some fresh cotton candy. It will put you in a better mood to talk to the owners, even if you are still unhappy with having us here."

"Now see here, miss—"

She pleaded with him sweetly. "Indulge me, sir, won't you?" She switched on the machine, which began to hum. "Indulge yourself."

The woman suddenly produced a box of sugar. Pink crystals poured down the spout at the center of the machine's cylinder.

"You've been living alone for so long. How many years has it been since Mae died?"

"I, huh?" Bragg's feeling of dislocation returned. Perhaps his initial shock at the woman's appearance had boomeranged. Certainly, it seemed hotter. And the sweet smell was starting to become sickening. And was she talking about Mae?

"When's the last time you had dessert, or even a piece of hard candy? Or anything sweet?" The woman held up a long, white paper cone. Then she pressed another button on the machine. The tumbler began to spin. Pink threads appeared in the drum. The Old Man watched mutely, aware of sweat beading on his forehead. For the first time since his youth, he was feeling the heat, noticing the weather.

The woman plunged the cone into the drum and began to twirl it. As she deftly flicked her wrist, cotton candy started to gather on the cone. The Old Man could swear the machine was producing pink sparks as well. Before he could make sense of this, she held up a large pink puff of cotton candy, as if presenting him with a bouquet of pink roses.

"It can't help but cheer you up, Mr. Bragg."

He took it mutely. It sure did look good to him. Better than he'd ever seen cotton candy. It almost glowed, even in the harsh glare of the July sun.

The woman took his arm again.

"Here, let's walk while you eat. Everything will be fine. The owners, I'm sure, are anxious to meet you and will try their best to make you happy."

They resumed walking toward the back of the carnival.

The Old Man took his first bite of the cotton candy. It tasted even better than it looked. Soft. Perfectly sweet. It melted into a sweet liquor in his mouth, which he swallowed slowly in order to savor the taste. Then he greedily bit into the cotton candy a second time. This mouthful he gulped down quickly in order to get to the next one. Each bite was a starburst in his mouth, like he was eating sweet caviar.

As he gobbled up the cotton candy, the woman beside him continued to smile in her bland, effortless way. The Old Man took no notice. A tent appeared before them. Above the entrance was a handwritten sign: Employees Only. The Old Man was too enthralled by his sugary delicacy to care about much else. Soon he had eaten all of the cotton candy. His lips and chin were pink with melted sugar. Less and less aware of himself, the Old Man sucked on the paper cone to get every last bit of sugar from it. Soon, the paper cone itself fell apart from the wetness of his saliva. Dropping it to the dusty ground, he ran his tongue over as much of his lips and chin as he could reach.

"Here we are," the woman sang out, leading him through the tent opening.

The inside of the tent was as dark as the Old Man's mind had become. And he was lost in that darkness, despite the now overwhelming sensation that everything had turned bright and pink and sweet. He stood inside the tent, with a slack smile on his face, seeing nothing but pink.

Out of the darkness, a strange, deep voice floated.

"You have done well," it said. "Put him with the others."

"Yes, sire," the woman answered.

Feeling a gentle tug on his arm, the Old Man willingly followed the woman toward the back of the tent, where they both disappeared into the darkness.

9

That evening, Lenore found herself on her way toward Ione's apartment, in what amounted to a gallows walk for her self-respect. In her one-room dorm room after class, she had devised a plan to get closer to Dimitri. Soon after 9 P.M. she found herself walking down the bar-lined street just off campus. The smell of beermud reminded her of Dimitri. Her mind suggested turning back then, but her body continued moving unfalteringly ahead.

Like the *Titanic* toward the iceberg.

With her legs seemingly on autopilot, her mind railed strongly against the mission at hand. *It's okay if you think you're a loser,* an inner voice screamed. *Even Mia can know that. And heck, let's throw in Dimitri as a bonus.*

But does anyone outside of that privileged circle need to know?

Turn back! Turn back now!

The voice seemed to emanate from her head and echo off the storefronts of the faux-Colonial shopping village just beyond bar row. The shops were dark now, the street deserted. Even the homeless that normally camped in doorways and alleys after hours were absent. Lenore walked along the curb in case there were any hidden in the shadows, ready to jump out at her.

Streetlights shining on the broad windows broadcast Lenore's progress like a street full of flat-screen televisions. She sneaked a look out of the corner of her eye. The images didn't portray her as a soldier marching toward destiny. The heavy night air once again weighing on her hair and clothes, she looked more like a shambling, postapocalyptic zombie.

She sighed but did not slow.

Swallowing hard, she told the voice inside her, *Ione will understand. In fact, I bet she* won't *understand, and that will make things much easier.*

Her classmate Ione wasn't the brightest bulb in the pack. She was quiet and gentle, with a perpetual faraway look. In short, she was a total space case.

And space cases tended to be kind, because it takes too much effort to be otherwise. And their retention isn't the best either.

So, Lenore thought to herself, *when I ask her to swap husbands with me so I can have Dimitri, whether she agrees or not, it'll be with a faint, sweet smile and an empty blink of the eyes.*

Lenore was banking on the fact that, at the very least, Ione couldn't muster the intellectual focus to be a bitch about the situation.

With a sudden roar and the blare of a powerful stereo, a muscle car zoomed past and screeched around the corner ahead. Tangled in her thoughts about Ione and her confusion over the mysterious thunder, Lenore nearly lost her balance and fell over. By the time she regained her focus, the car had disappeared.

Picking up the pace, Lenore "quick-time harched" toward her humiliation. She soon turned onto Ione's block, where well-kept forties-era row houses faced each other from across a tree-lined street. Lenore sighed. It was perfect. Idyllic. Romantic.

And just the type of cozy environment she imagined sharing with Dimitri.

Sure, she was poor, with no car, living in nondescript campus housing, and he was a haughty rich kid living in his parents' mansion in the exclusive area of town. But this is where they could meet in the middle. She could rise above her current station. And he could descend from Olympus and learn how to be mortal.

Ione's building loomed up on her left. It was a three-story brownstone that would have looked right at home on New York's Upper West Side. Light shone from the windows of the top floor. Ione was home.

Lenore paused before the stairs leading to the brownstone's front door. Between her nervousness and the dense air, she was panting. Behind her, she could hear the ticking of a cooling car engine. Across the street was the muscle car that had zoomed past her. The sight of it fed her rising panic.

Something metallic rattled just beyond the car—a lone homeless guy, pushing a shopping cart full of recyclable cans and bottles, plastic bags tied to its sides hanging like tumors. He stopped to watch her. She recognized him immediately as Ass-Face, the one-eyed vagrant. Even from across the street, even the notion of his empty, shriveled socket unnerved her.

To escape his cyclopean stare, Lenore whipped herself back around and marched up the stone stairs. She reached up to buzz Ione's flat but noticed that the front door was wedged open by an old newspaper.

Taking a deep breath, she entered the brownstone. Once in the foyer, she turned to look back at the street. Ass-Face continued to stare at her.

Using her foot, she dragged the newspaper into the foyer and pulled the door tightly shut.

The floor was constructed of old-style, octagonal white tiles with an evenly spaced scattering of single black tiles. The air was stuffy and smelled of elderly residents. As she expected, the building was a walk-up. With one more fortifying deep breath, she gripped the dark, lacquered-wood railing and started up the stairs.

She kept a steady pace up each flight of stairs. The building was silent around her, as if the thick air dampened all sound. And as she ascended, the air in the stairwell just became denser and more humid.

I hope she has air-conditioning, Lenore thought. *Or we'll suffocate before we're done talking.*

Just off the landing of the third floor was an unmarked door. Beyond, down the hallway, another door stood open. Lenore paused momentarily at the unmarked door, then decided to head toward the open door, in front of which lay a welcome mat. Holding onto the door frame to maintain balance, Lenore leaned into the apartment.

"Hello? Ione?"

Two things struck Lenore immediately. One was that the place did not have air-conditioning. She had a moment of satisfaction thinking this meant Ione had less of an advantage over her than she had thought. In the next moment, the overwhelming smell of ammonia hit her.

Lenore coughed and called out again, but no one answered. Even so, she thought she heard movement inside the apartment.

She stepped into the front hallway, which opened up on a spacious living room to the left. To the right, a hallway ran back in the direction of the stairs. The living room was empty, although the TV was on. In green digital letters, the word MUTE floated on the screen. A vacuum cleaner stood in the center of the room, its cord running across the floor to a wall outlet. The entire room looked neat and tidy, as if it had just been straightened.

Just then, Lenore heard a soft thump from the back of the apartment.

"Ione?" she called out again. And again, there was no answer.

Lenore entered the hallway, moving toward the sound she had heard. A doorway stood on her left several feet ahead, and she could see another door at the end of the hallway.

Tentatively, Lenore peered into the doorway on her left.

A wave of ammonia odor hit her. Nausea was the next wave to wash over her, but not because of the chemical smell. The sparkling white kitchen contained a dark stain of horror.

Ione lay on the floor, facing the ceiling, her eyes rolled up into her head. Out of her mouth swelled a black tongue. There was no blood. But from the expression in her face, Ione had died a horrible death.

So overwhelmed by the sight, and by the stifling, chemical-tinged air, Lenore could not scream.

She quickly surveyed the room. The dead girl wore yellow rubber gloves on both hands, one in a death grip around a crushed canister of powdered cleanser. On the counter, many bottles of cleaners had been knocked over, their contents spilling all over the place and forming a cloudy blue lake between the sink and

Ione's body. Like an island in the center of the lake lay a bag of flour. It had fallen, apparently from the sink, and had burst upon the ground.

Lenore staggered backwards into the hallway. She had to call the police. But not from here. She couldn't remain with Ione's corpse for another moment. She would just close the front door behind her, and Ione would be just fine until the police came.

"Lenore."

Dimitri appeared in the hallway. He stood between her and the way out of Ione's apartment. She noticed immediately he was covered in green and white powder.

"What have you done?"

She had expected to find Dimitri here—it was his car that had careened by her and was now parked across the street. But she hadn't expected to find Ione dead.

"I haven't done anything," he told her, speaking slowly. "Now calm down."

His own unnatural calm only made her more nervous. He stepped toward her, hands up. They were the only part of him not coated with powder.

"Stay away from me!" Lenore yelled and fled back down the hallway.

"Lenore, wait!" He came after her.

Lenore rushed through the bedroom door at the end of the hall and slammed it shut behind her. Dimitri's footsteps pounded down the hallway, just behind her. She flipped the dead bolt, locking the door just as he reached it. Almost immediately, the doorknob started rattling, and he banged on the door.

"Open up, Lenore!" he called out. "I'm not going to hurt you."

Sniffling, Lenore just backed up against Ione's bed. The doorknob jerked hard to one side, and then the entire door bowed inward as Dimitri threw his shoulder into it. Despite the dead bolt, the door wouldn't hold for very long.

"Open the door, you bitch!" Dimitri called out. "We have to talk about this."

"What did you do to Ione?!"

"Just listen to me!" Dimitri called out. With a grunt, he shouldered the door once more. Paint cracked around the door's upper hinge.

Frantically, Lenore searched the room. She didn't relish jumping out a third-story window, but she resolved to do it if Dimitri broke down the door. Then she found the second door, next to the closet's mirrored sliding doors.

Behind her, Dimitri hit the door again, and this time, the upper hinge pulled away from the doorframe by a quarter of an inch.

She threw the second door open and stepped out into the outer hallway, near the landing. This was the unmarked door she had passed on her way in. She ran down the first flight of steps, making it to the next landing, when she heard a huge crash from above.

Dimitri had broken down Ione's bedroom door.

Screaming, Lenore plunged down the next flight of stairs.

"Get the fuck back here!" Dimitri roared and came after her.

Halfway down the final flight of stairs, Lenore fell, tumbling down the stairs and landing on the hard white tile of the entranceway. She lay there for a moment, stunned.

Dimitri appeared at the landing above her and took the final steps in one jump. But he misjudged his height, and his forehead struck the overhang from the upper level. He cried out in pain and fell backwards onto the stairs.

Lenore flipped onto her front, pushed herself to her feet, and headed out the front door.

Behind her, the door had barely closed before Dimitri, groaning in pain, flung it open again. He gave chase as Lenore ran screaming back toward the Colonial shopping village.

Ass-Face, who hadn't moved since Lenore had entered the building, watched the chase with his remaining eye.

Lenore's voice ran out about the time she found herself in front of the hardware store. The windows now broadcast a woman in abject terror, not a dull, shambling zombie. A sharp pain in her chest caused her to stop. She could no longer move, no longer breathe. She was leaning against a recessed doorway when Dimitri caught up with her a moment later.

She shrieked and collapsed against the door, landing on her butt. Dimitri likewise collapsed in front of her, his chest heaving.

"What is your problem?" he gasped. "I said I wouldn't hurt you."

"That's what people say before they hurt you." Lenore was catching her breath but trying to pretend not to. Without looking down, she started to visualize her foot kicking Dimitri in the crotch.

"Move over," Dimitri said suddenly and shoved her aside. They sat next to each other on a short step. His shoulder touched hers. She could smell him, the heat and sweat rising from him. Suddenly, she was not so afraid.

"I don't care what you think, or what it looked like, I didn't kill Ione, you got that?" He was still panting, and talking seemed to make things worse. "You got that?" He was looking at her now, demanding a response.

"Okay," she replied. "But what happened?"

"I don't know."

"What were you doing there, anyway?"

Dimitri snorted some exhausted laughter. "To get a divorce, actually."

"What?"

"I was gonna have her ditch me so I could get Mia for this stupid parenting assignment."

Lenore's heart sank listening to him, but she tried not to show her disappointment.

"It occurred to me when Aiden dropped the class. If I could talk Ione into it, then that would pave the way for Mia and me to be together. I went up to talk to her about it, and . . ."

His voice hitched, then trailed off entirely. He remained silent for nearly a minute before saying, "Anyway, I found her that way, I swear."

"What about that stuff all over you?" Lenore asked.

He shrugged. "I checked her out, hoping she was still alive. I guess this crap got on me then." He stared off into the distance. He laughed briefly again. "Wow. Our 'kid' around all those chemicals. Would have been dangerous if it had been a real baby."

Lenore turned to him sharply. "Ione's dead, Dimitri. How can you make jokes?"

"Hey, it's either laugh or cry, ya know?"

They both fell silent for a moment. Then he brushed his pants off and stood, groaning in pain as he did so.

"My head and my back are going to be so fucked up tomorrow," he said. Then he reached down to Lenore. "Come on."

She hesitated before taking his hand and standing.

"Where to?"

"Back to Ione's," he told her.

Lenore pulled away from him. "I don't want to."

"We *have* to go back there, sweetcakes. As you pointed out, Ione's dead. So we have to report it to the police. And we have to be together, because our fingerprints and footprints are all over that place. We're each other's alibis."

Reluctantly, she agreed to return. As they rounded the corner she noticed an orange glow coming from Ione's apartment.

She pointed up. "Were there any candles burning or anything like that?"

Dimitri saw what she was looking at. His jaw dropped.

"Oh shit, a fire. Come on!"

The got up to the apartment to find nothing. No orange glow. No smoke. Nothing. No fire.

Stranger still: no Ione.

The kitchen was sparkling and empty. The bottles had been removed from the counter. The powder and liquid on the floors had been cleaned. The yellow rubber gloves lay neatly draped on the edge of the sink. It was as if Ione had risen from the floor, finished cleaning while they'd been gone, then had vanished into thin air.

In the living room, the TV had been turned off, and the vacuum cleaner cord had been neatly wound into its handle. Only the rent bedroom door prevented Lenore from thinking they had gone completely nuts. But someone had been here. The door had been shut, the paint chips and wood splinters swept away.

Lenore followed Dimitri around the apartment in a daze. Everything looked utterly normal. Not sure what else to do, they left the apartment.

They walked to his car silently and leaned against it.

"Let me take you home," he said dully.

Sluggishly, Lenore tugged at the passenger door until Dimitri finally unlocked it.

"What do we do now?" she asked as he started the car.

"There's nothing *to* do," he said. "I know what you saw. What I saw. But it ain't there for anyone else to see."

He let the car idle while they talked.

"But she was dead, Dimitri. Wasn't she?"

He shook his head. "I don't know anymore. I could have sworn." He revved the engine, as if it helped him think. "It's not like anyone could have come in, taken the body and cleaned the place up in the short time we were gone."

Lenore agreed that it was impossible. But the other scenario was that Ione had played an elaborate—and tasteless—joke on them. Somehow, that seemed even less likely.

As she pondered this, Lenore spotted Ass-Face's shopping cart on the sidewalk just ahead of them. He was nowhere in sight.

10

For The Shower Tones, trouble began the next morning, midway through their delivery of "Coney Island Baby," bare-chested and writhing, onto the rehearsal room floor. Their voices trailed off at the violent pounding at the door. With a sigh, Buddy rose from his knees as the other Shower Tones instinctively cowered together. They attempted to rebutton their shirts, only to find that most of the buttons had popped off when they'd torn them open.

"Snaps next time, guys," Quincy whispered. The others nodded in agreement and just pulled their shirts closed as best they could.

Buddy opened the door, and immediately a blur pushed into the room, yelling.

"That's it! You guys are gone!" A pudgy man with an oily bald head nearly trampled Buddy. The man stopped, sized up the group, who stood clutching their shirts closed, and then whirled back at him.

Buddy was fascinated by how the man turned from *within*, followed by the looser, fatter parts of his body moments later.

"This is a *music* building, Mr. Bragg." He drew out the word *music* so that it sounded like "meee-oooooooosic." The man's chest heaved with rage and the effort to sustain it. "Your pathetic efforts at barber-shop at least had some grounding in a respected musi-cal tradition. But I will *not* allow the resources of this school, this music"—meeeooooooosic—"school, to be wasted on such nonsense!"

Buddy took a beat and looked at his shoe. He liked to take a beat. This often put others off their guard. In this case, it would give Professor Farber a chance to calm down. Farber had never been a fan of Buddy's. The man was a die-hard classical musician. His was a world of Mozart and Stravinsky and Rachmaninoff. Most of his record collection still consisted of antique 78s. Farber took a dim view of any instruments that required electrical power.

Professor Farber had been born several hundred years too late, and he took out his frustration on every-one else.

Quincy, mistaking Buddy's pause for an awkward silence, leaped into the gap.

"We're, uh, students here, Professor Farber," Quincy said. "We have a right to use these facilities."

The others instinctively shrank back from him, in

order to avoid bloodstains if Farber suddenly ripped him to pieces.

"If I want your opinion, Peterson, I'll ask Mr. Bragg here for it," he said without turning around. Then he looked directly at Buddy, who was now cultivating a slightly bored stare.

"Your previous efforts have always perched precariously on the razor edge of the rules, Mr. Bragg. But this time, you've fallen off this edge." Farber lumbered closer. Buddy could smell his breath. The spectre of a recently deceased liver-and-onions breakfast hovered between them. "Your current endeavor requires no instruments and involves a musical style"—his smooth face wrinkled slightly in profound disgust—"not recognized by this school's curriculum. Ergo, you have no need or claim to this school's resources for your questionable little social club."

Buddy arranged a slight smirk on his face. They were sunk, so it wouldn't change their fate. He'd just get more satisfaction from the outcome.

"No need to beat around the bush, Professor Farber. We're all adults. What're you trying to say?"

Behind Farber, the eyes of The Shower Tones grew wide with fear. The entire group took a full step backwards and huddled closer together.

As expected, Buddy's insolence set off a series of tremors in Farber's thick body. His fists clenched and unclenched at his sides. The red in his bald pate deepened. The oily sheen became more pronounced. Buddy shifted his weight from one leg to the other and absently scratched his bared left nipple as he waited for Vesuvius to erupt.

"You *freak!!*" the professor finally yelled, saliva spraying from his mouth. Then he turned and wagged a pudgy finger at the rest of the group. "You're *all* freaks! Get out of my building. Now. And never, ever, *ever* come back!"

Buddy stepped aside as Farber barreled past him and threw open the door. Outside in the hall, students had gathered to listen to the row. Most were smiling in triumph, obviously eager to be rid of The Shower Tones.

Strolling casually over to the door, Buddy winked at the crowd outside before pushing the door closed between them. Before it had closed completely, he noticed an older woman among the students. She was dressed like Agent Scully from *The X-Files* and wore sunglasses. *Weird,* he thought mildly. She looked very out of place. He forgot about her the instant he turned back to his friends.

"All great artists were persecuted in their day," he told them grandly.

After a moment of silence, Quincy raised a hand to speak.

"What are we gonna do now?" he asked.

"I mean, this was fresh and all, you know," Wes said as he buttoned his shirt.

Buddy noticed he was missing no buttons and took a mental note: *Wes has experience ripping his shirt from his body*.

"You guys are chill," Wes continued, "but, like, it's not like we need to do this."

Trevin nodded in agreement, evidently shamed by his feelings.

"Too bad," Thomas said. "I was down with this. But I gots to agree."

"Stupid. Very stupid," Uni chimed in curtly.

"You guys," Buddy said, his voice dripping with disappointment. "We're having fun, right? You need any other incentive?"

The rest of The Shower Tones shifted uncomfortably in place and looked everywhere in the room but at Buddy. He shook his head and clucked at them.

"Guys. Dudes. *Bros!* Look. For classes, you gotta do homework and turn it in. Right? And all this goes toward graduation, something you're expected to do. Then get a job, get married, make partner, get a bonus for exceeding your quota, whatever. So you got goals. And you're given goals. But it's not *all* about goals, man. It's not just about putting a coin in the machine and getting out a gumball. Maybe a good goal is not to have a goal, at least for some things." Buddy spread out his hands, inviting any sort of response.

"Well, ahem, sure, Buddy," Quincy finally said, raising his hand. "But I mean, if this is what happens, if we get kicked out of the music building and become jokes, I mean, is that fun?"

"What does the world outside this room have to do with any fun we have in this room?" Buddy asked.

"Weh-weh-well, we did get kicked out cuh-cuz no one luh-luh-liked us out there," Trevin pointed out reluctantly.

Buddy nodded slightly to concede the point. He looked at the others, inviting additional comments.

"I am here to learn," Uni barked in his harsh, deep voice. "Not sing. I join to make friends. Now I lose friends because of singing."

"What're you talking about?" Buddy gestured to the rest of the group. "You got seven friends right there. That's a lot of friends, and I mean *real* friends, in today's world."

Uni just looked at the others dubiously.

"If you ask me," Ty whined, "and I know you wouldn't, because you never do, we're just at a point of diminishing returns. Even if we could rehearse, which I just can't see in our dorm rooms or off-campus apartments, where would we perform? I mean, what's the point?"

"*That's* my point!" Buddy shouted, pointing suddenly at Ty with one hand and tapping his nose with the index finger of the other hand. "That we have no point. But that we share in our pointlessness!"

Everyone looked away from him again. He could see that it wasn't sinking in. Professor Farber's attack had galvanized them against Buddy's usual charms. They were scared and embarrassed, and at the moment all looked like a group of skittish horses. Wes was the first to bolt.

"Much love to you guys," said the baritone as he stepped forward. "But boy band music is so, nineties, you know what I mean? Most of those guys are older than us, anyway." He thrust his fist forward, and Buddy butted it with his. "We'll chill sometime." He strode to the door, adding "Peace out," before he left.

Buddy turned back to the group.

"I look up on Internet," said Uni brusquely. "Ninety-Eight Degrees already do 'Coney Island Baby.' " After a slight bow, he, too, left the room.

"Wes's right," Thomas said. "They're all bustin' up and going solo anyway." He offered Buddy a high five and left with a "Hang loose, bro!"

Trevin simply said, "I'm sorry," and skulked from the room.

"I guess we'll just have to live with being pussies," offered Flutie, shrugging his broad, meaty shoulders and squeezing through the rehearsal room doorway.

Ty left two steps behind Flutie, as if attempting to hide in the first tenor's wake. He didn't say a word. Only Quincy remained.

"Et tu Brute?"

Quincy smiled. "No, I haven't 'et' yet. Let's grab some lunch." He clapped Buddy on the shoulder, but Buddy didn't move. "What? Buddy Bragg feeling sorry for himself? Good thing the guys aren't here to see this."

"I've had friends move on, but never had them walk out on me." Buddy continued to stare at the space The Shower Tones had occupied only minutes before.

"That was Farber's fault and you know it," Quincy told him. "The Shower Tones might be washed up, but you're not."

"Of course I'm not. And I don't think The Shower Tones are either." Buddy turned and placed his hands on Quincy's shoulders. "I really *did* dream that boy band thing. This isn't over, not for me, not for you, not for them."

Quincy searched Buddy's face for any sign of the usual Buddy white noise. He found none. Gently, he lifted Buddy's hands from his shoulders.

"You'll have to tell me about this dream. And what you were on when you had it." He laughed, but Buddy did not. "Anyway, let's grab some lunch."

"You go on ahead," Buddy said, staring again into the room. The outline of the group seemed burned into his vision, as if he had looked into a cluster of bright lights. "I'll meet you at the Student Union in a couple minutes."

Quincy nodded. Buddy didn't like the look of concern in his friend's face. It meant he was too naked right now. That's why he wanted Quincy to go on ahead; he needed to collect himself.

"See you in a few," Quincy said.

"Now what?" Buddy asked the purple ghosts of the friends who had just abandoned him.

As if in answer, Buddy heard the door rattle behind him. He turned toward it. With a quiet scraping, a red piece of paper slid under the door from the hallway.

Ignoring the card, Buddy threw the door open. No one was there. The hallway was deserted. With one last glance, in case someone, anyone, came into view, Buddy returned to the rehearsal room.

He picked up the red paper, a piece of card stock about half the size of a piece of typing paper. Printed on it were the words:

The perpetuals
present
A Fun Faire!
Rides! Midway Games!
Laugh-in-the-Dark
plus!
The perpetuals' Magick Mirror Maze
And our very special
cavalcade of oddities side show!
(This free pass good for up to 8 people)

The lettering was an Old English type, very thick and black. Buddy scratched the *P* in Perpetuals, and black ink chipped off, wedging under his fingernail. The entire card apparently had been produced by an old-fashioned printing press, with ink-rollers and woodblock letters, rather than on a laser or ink-jet printer. A lot of work.

The back of the card contained two important pieces of information. One was directions, which placed the Fun Faire just off the freeway on the edge of town. These were printed in a simple, readable block type. Below, however, was a curious handwritten note, scrawled in a florid script. Buddy's jaw nearly dropped. The message was an invitation: an invitation to fulfill a dream. *The* dream. His nimble mind figured out how to make this happen almost instantly.

Buddy stuffed the carnival announcement into his back pocket and ran to meet Quincy.

11

After a night filled with dreams that made Orson Welles's filmed version of Kafka's *The Trial* look like an episode of Barney the Purple Dinosaur, Lenore returned to Waman's Human Sexuality class. From his seat, Dimitri gave her a barely imperceptible nod. Ironic, she thought, that it took an apparent murder to make him notice her again. When Ione appeared in class, their tenuous connection would probably be severed, she thought sadly. Before taking her seat next to Mia, she scanned the room. So far, no Ione.

"What's up with you?" Mia asked her, elbowing her in the shoulder. "Your legs are pumping like you're in a spinning class!"

Lenore looked down at her legs, which had unconsciously been quivering since she sat down.

"Sorry," she said, and willed her legs still. "I just had a venti coffee instead of a grande this morning."

"Whatever," Mia said and cuddled up against Zander as Professor Waman cleared his throat to signal the start of class. The room settled down quickly.

"Apparently, some of you are having trouble handling the assignment," he said. He shuffled papers on the podium, making marks on the class list. "Three students dropped our little class since yesterday." He looked up from his papers with a dark smile. "Mr. Carlton," he said. "Please stand."

Lenore looked across the room. Dimitri stood with great effort and seemed ready to bolt from the room.

"My condolences," Professor Waman said. "But it appears you have lost a wife in the process. Apparently, Ms. Delacorte couldn't stand the heat and got out of the kitchen."

Dimitri staggered back and dropped into his seat. Lenore let out a small gasp. Dimitri was trying very hard not to look her way.

"She has dropped the class, leaving you without a wife or child. Imagine that." Professor Waman turned to the rest of the class. "We're two for two, ladies and gentlemen. Luckily for you," he said, addressing Dimitri once more, "there is a single mother in this class who could use a good husband. Lacking that, there is you."

"No!" Lenore whispered under her breath.

"No!" protested Mia in a louder voice.

"I'll be pairing you with Ms. Miller for the remainder of the assignment."

Dimitri's shocked expression gave way to one of triumph. He turned toward Lenore and looked right through her to Mia. Whatever they had witnessed the night before had evidently evaporated from his mind. Lenore could hear their delicate bond snapping in her mind and in her heart. She slumped in her seat as Mia rose from hers in protest.

"This isn't fair!" she raged. "You can't change the assignment on me twice in two days!"

"Your protest is duly noted, Ms. Miller," he said perfunctorily. "However, you two, as well as the rest of you, will be expected to sit together during class in order to present a coherent family unit and to deliver your reports."

"But Professor—," Mia began again, but Waman silenced her immediately.

"Part of life is rolling with the punches, Ms. Miller," Waman told her. "And you'll just have to learn to roll with this . . ."

Waman's face suddenly went pale. For a moment, his mouth simply hung open as he stared toward the back of the lecture hall. His normally impassive face showed more expression than it had in the last two days. With effort, he regained his composure. In the upper doorway stood a woman wearing a dark business suit and sunglasses. She seemed to wait until she had everyone's attention before descending toward the podium and Professor Waman. In her hands she held a stack of red cards.

"May I help you?" Waman finally asked, very clearly on edge. He sounded like a bank teller cooperating with a bank robber until he could surreptitiously trigger the silent alarm.

The woman addressed Waman in a bright and cheery voice. "I am an emissary of the Perpetuals, Professor."

Despite her good-natured tone, Professor Waman's body went rigid, as if he were preparing to bolt from the room.

"I come with free passes for your students to the Perpetuals' Fun Faire!"

She held up the stack of red cards as if they were gold bars. But Waman's flat, wary response sharply contrasted the woman's almost artificial cheeriness.

"This is a classroom, Ms. . . . whatever your name is. I'll have to ask you to leave."

The woman finally reached the lower level of the lecture hall. Incredibly, she then ignored Waman and addressed the class directly.

"The Fun Faire is an old-style carnival, complete with rides, Laugh-in-the-Dark fun house, Magick Mirror Maze and, best of all, a sideshow of exotic part-human creatures from all over the world called the Cavalcade of Oddities!"

Lenore got the distinct impression she had found herself in some surreal infomercial.

At his podium, Waman began to shake with anger. The woman continued to ignore him.

"We're new in town, not officially opening until tomorrow, but we would like to extend an opportunity for *you*"—she pointed toward the students—"to preview the Fun Faire for free! Then maybe you'll tell your friends. *And* families."

"Now see here, Miss . . . ," Waman began. His ponytail shook with rage.

The woman finally turned her head toward him and continued talking.

"Yes, the Fun Faire is a perfect place to bring the family! I'm going to leave this stack of free passes on this table. Come pick them up after class, and we look forward to seeing you at the Fun Faire tonight!"

She placed the red cards on the lab table and turned back to the class with a broad smile. Then, with a jovial nod to the professor, the woman marched back up the stairs and out of the classroom.

No one spoke for a full minute. No one was quite sure what they had just seen. The professor removed the top card from the stack the woman had left and examined it, huffing as he tried to calm himself down. He turned it over, his anger turning to curiosity. Then another knowing smile.

Lenore was coming to prefer his stone face. His smiles held reminders of her Kafka dreams.

"Um, what is that?" a student finally asked.

"An invitation," Waman said. "One we would be rude to refuse." He folded the card in half and placed it in his breast pocket. Then he took the stack from the desk and thrust it at Perry. "Pass these across and back."

The students broke out in whispered conversations as they passed the cards through the lecture hall.

"Ladies and gentlemen," Professor Waman announced, "tonight has just been designated Family Night at this Fun Faire. Class is dismissed until eight-thirty this evening, when we will all meet at the entrance to this carnival. Everyone will be expected to arrive paired with your spouse and with your child conveyed by some acceptable means."

Many in the class protested immediately.

"Very good," he said, ignoring them. "I will see you all at eight-thirty sharp."

Waman gathered papers from the podium and retreated to his office. Students knocked at his door to ask what exactly was expected of them, but he didn't answer.

"What is that guy's problem?" Mia huffed after throwing her bag of flour into a booth at the Student Union. She threw herself in after.

"Careful!" Lenore said, sitting across from Mia.

"If I bust it, I'll just go to a grocery store and pick up a new one. Jeez!" But she lifted the beige bag from the seat and placed it carefully on the table before her. "There. Happy?"

Zander slid into the booth next to her.

"Calm down, honey."

Mia crossed her arms and growled.

"Um, tell you what," Lenore said. "I mean, if it would make it easier on you, we can trade. At least you wouldn't have to deal with Dimitri. We can talk to Waman and—"

Mia started groaning before Lenore had finished. "Focus, sweetie. One thing at a time. My anger, *then* your pathetic obsession."

Lenore leaned back as if Mia had slapped her in the face. Even Zander was taken aback.

"Hey, that's so not cool."

Mia slumped back in her seat.

"This is bullshit," she said, mostly to herself. Then she turned to Lenore. "Ya know I don't mean it."

Lenore had already begun to slide out of the booth.

"That's not the same thing as 'I'm sorry,' " she said, standing.

"Look, I'm sorry, but—"

" 'Sorry' stopped cutting it awhile ago, Mia. You should try stopping yourself before you say and do things you end up sorry for." Lenore began to shake, right as Dimitri appeared.

"Hey Lenore," he said, noticing her distress. "How long can you go like that before the batteries wear out?"

Lenore collapsed on the seat and buried her face in her arms, fighting back the sobs.

"Don't be a dick, Dimbulb." Mia touched Lenore's arm to comfort her, but Lenore pulled away.

"Anyway," he said, turning Lenore off in his mind like a light switch. "How's my wife?"

"Stuff it," answered Mia. "In case you hadn't heard, Zander and I are engaged for real. I wouldn't take moronic class assignments too seriously."

"I'll take what I can get," Dimitri said. "I'm a patient man. How 'bout I pick you up at 7 P.M. tonight in the mighty Mustang?"

"Uh, how about not?" Mia said, rolling her eyes.

Zander started to massage Mia's shoulders. To everyone's surprise, he said, "Maybe you should."

Lenore raised her head, her sobs subsiding. Mia looked at Zander like he had just suggested experimenting with bestiality.

"Look, I'll take Lenore, and the four of us can meet up at the park. If Waman sees us arrive in our assigned pairs, it'll help our grades. Once we're there we'll just get through the evening as painlessly as possible." Then he looked Dimitri dead in the eye. "And afterwards, it's over. It is what it is."

Dimitri stared back, considering his answer.

"I'm supposed to go with Dimbulb?" Mia asked, her voice rising.

"We'll be together once we get there," Zander assured her. "All of us."

Mia sighed in resignation. "All right. As long as *you*," she said directly to Dimitri, "know that this is just for the assignment. Afterwards, you get off my back."

"Done," Dimitri said with a sharp nod. "Double date's better than no date."

"It's *not* a date!" Mia roared.

"Whatever." Dimitri winked at her and ran a finger quickly down Lenore's spine. "Later gator."

Lenore sat bolt upright in her seat. His fingers had left a wake of goose bumps.

Mia turned on Zander as soon as Dimitri left. "What did you do that for?"

"Let's just say that spending tonight all together would be a good reality check. For all of us." He looked at Lenore oddly. "Maybe this would be good for her," he said. "Give her a chance to really get to know him. Figure out if he's really worth the trouble."

Lenore's face grew hotter, an embarrassed flush warming the goose bumps.

"Okay fine," Mia said. "That's plan B. But plan A is this. Once we get there, you and me will stick together, and all we'll talk about is our wedding plans, and how fabulous it will be, and how happy we'll be together and how many kids we're gonna have. Real kids, not these stupid things." She swatted the bag of flour. "Dimbulb can't help but get the picture."

"Right," Zander said.

"And who knows?" Mia said, looking up at Lenore with an evil grin. "Maybe Mother Teresa here is right, and your underachieving little dream will come true!"

"Maybe," Lenore said slowly, ignoring Mia's sarcasm.

Maybe, somehow, Dimitri *would* be hers before the night was over.

12

ater that midsummer afternoon, Lenore struggled over what to wear for the evening. Clearly, Dimitri was attracted by Mia's edgier and more expensive fashions. Cloning Mia's wardrobe was not an option, but neither was remaining with classic, and classically ineffective, Lenore frilly-and-dowdy. But how to upgrade without buying new clothes that she simply couldn't afford?

Think, Lenore, think. This thought allowed her to identify her problem: she *thought* too much. Mia, on the other hand, possessed a sort of preternatural fashion sense that went beyond genetic. Anything she bought and wore seemed to adapt itself to her image and her body.

The only thing Lenore thought would adapt to her own body was a parachute.

And so she grasped handfuls of hangers from her closet and threw them, clothes and all, on the bed. Like a three-card monte dealer on a New York street corner, she arranged and rearranged tops, skirts and footwear over and over again. But unlike a street hustler, she never felt close to winning her own game.

On the other side of campus, Uni sat coping. Some people dealt with stress by gorging on food. Others shopped. He programmed. Since the rehearsal broke up, he had been sitting for hours in front of his computer, swimming in machine language. Its rigidity and logic made him feel safe. Each subroutine was a predictable cause-and-effect scenario, which was something he couldn't say about his life, no matter how satisfying at times, as an acolyte of Buddy Bragg's.

On the opposite side of his dorm room's common area, a place that in most suites approximated a living room with a television and video game system, sat Uni's roommate, Tak, also a Japanese exchange student. The two had met as dorm mates only a month ago. Tak also sat before a computer monitor, also working through a programming assignment. But for him, programming was breathing. He seemed to think if he stopped, he would die. Surrounded by books and manuals on a wide variety of computer-related technical issues, their common room looked more like an IS department than a living area.

Tak had been hard at work, as usual, when Uni had returned from rehearsal. Aside from a brief bow when Uni had entered the room, they had not acknowledged each other the entire time, which also was the norm. Neither played music while they worked. Their dorm

room had all the atmosphere of a library. Or a mau-
soleum. Uni had tried playing music after he had fallen
in with Buddy, but Tak had told him brusquely that he
found it a distraction from studies. Ever polite, Uni had
obliged him, and a cone of silence had enveloped the
room ever since.

Unfortunately, Uni's coping mechanism was faulty.
The sound of keyboard tapping for hours on end even-
tually made him feel like he was surrounded by evil
woodpeckers. Sighing loudly, he spun in his office
chair.

"Hey, Tak, do you want to see a movie later?" he
asked in Japanese.

Tak paused in his work but did not look back.
"American cinema is soft as baby food," he said sternly
and whipped the woodpeckers into a frenzy once more.

Uni sank in his chair. He should have known better.
Sighing, he turned back and raised his hands unwill-
ingly to the keyboard once more. Before he could
begin to type, the phone rang. Tak did not even pause
in his work; he never got calls on anything but the high-
tech cell phone he had brought from Japan.

Uni hesitated before answering the phone. Since
he'd arrived on campus, only members of The Shower
Tones had used this number. Not even his parents
called from Japan. No doubt it would be Quincy, begging on Buddy's behalf to return to the fold. No way, he
thought, then reached for the phone before Quincy
hung up.

His tenuous grasp on the English language made it hard for Uni to express emotion, especially over the phone. But the moment he heard Quincy's voice, he was overjoyed. And he said yes immediately to what Quincy asked, then hung up the phone.

Uni switched off his computer, grabbed his coat and left the dorm room without saying good-bye to Tak, whom he never saw again.

True to Lenore's assessment, Mia barely thought about clothes, other than the occasional label check. Even her consistent psuedo-punk style was not a conscious decision. Those kind of clothes seemed simply to gravitate toward her and onto her. And so while Lenore was losing her own three-card monte game, Mia won by not playing. Instead, she spent the afternoon planning her wedding with Zander.

Mother hadn't approved when she'd told her yesterday, but then, Mother rarely approved of anything she hadn't mulled carefully over a bottle of Ketel One.

No matter. Mia had her own bank account. She and Zander could live comfortably on the interest alone. Where they would live comfortably was the important issue to her. Only a few neighborhoods in Stratford were exclusive enough for her tastes. Her parents lived in one, Dimitri in the other. Proximity to either was highly undesirable. Zander's apartment, over a record store in the lower-rent end of the retail street near campus, was an option.

Puh. Leaze. Mia snorted laughter at her little joke. As a getaway from her parents, Zander's place served quite nicely. At least he had learned to wash on a weekly basis the three-hundred thread-count cotton sheets she had given him. But as for a long-term living arrangement? *Sorry folks, I just don't do squalor.*

The thought of squalor turned her thoughts from living arrangements to their honeymoon. A priority was some tropical, third-world country with both a favorable exchange rate and a resort environment utterly separate from the country's grubby, indigenous culture. The irony, she thought, was that due to economics, she could virtually ensure going to one of the poorest nations in the world and managing not to see even one dirt-smudged face. In America, by contrast, you couldn't walk without stepping on one, like ants.

Mia wrinkled her nose. What was she doing thinking about insects and bums when she had a wedding to plan? And she only had a few hours. Although the whats and wheres of her marriage to Zander might change in the long run, she wanted to have lots to talk about tonight at the Fun Faire.

Lots of fabulous details of her and Zander's future to rub in Dimitri's face.

Tonight might be fairly fun after all, Mia thought.

At the popular off-campus diner, Titus, Thomas ordered a garden salad at the counter. The waitress—and at a hard-lived fifty, she was a waitress in the old style, not a "server"—gave him an odd look and mumbled, "Whatever you want, honey." She had to speak up over the sound of burgers frying in the background. As he waited for his salad, Thomas looked around the diner, humming to himself.

He spied Trevin sitting alone in a far corner booth, staring down at a half-eaten meal. Thomas started to call out when he noticed that Trevin seemed to be listening to, or trying desperately to ignore, a group of students in the booth next to his. They were turned his way, speaking animatedly, though Thomas could not hear their words. They were a pretty average-looking group, four of them, of upper classmen. Black cases on the floor under their booth marked them as music students. Thomas identified two violins, a flute and a French horn by the shapes of the cases. The four shared a cruel and conspiratorial smile. He recognized bullies a mile away. And these were the worst kind: music school bullies.

One appeared to say something terribly amusing, and all four erupted in harsh laughter. Trevin continued to stare down at his meal, as if attempting to use heat vision to warm it up.

As Thomas watched, a ball of wadded-up napkin bounced off Trevin's face. He didn't even flinch.

Thomas had seen enough, and he rose from the service counter. Without saying a word, he approached the booths.

"Come on, sing us a song," said one of the bullies. "Sing for us, pretty boy!"

"Yeah, Barbra, sing us some 'Evergreen'!" said another.

Thomas clenched his fists. Once upon a time, he had been a bully of the more conventional and physical kind. But long ago, losing himself in the music of Luther Vandross, he had found the peace and the smoothness and had changed his ways.

But for the moment, these guys didn't need to know that.

"Sup," he said quietly in a voice that boomed nonetheless. Trevin looked up, and for a moment his lip trembled. He was about to burst into tears. The students at the table turned quickly as well.

"We wanna hear from the—oh shit." Upon seeing Thomas, the student instinctively reached for his violin case.

"Is that all you got to say? 'Oh shit'? You're hassling my buddy, and the best you can do is 'Oh shit'?" Thomas stood at the head of their table, blocking their exit. Each of the bully musicians had grabbed his instrument and now looked ready to bolt.

"We were just having fun," one said, desperately turning to Trevin. "We're cool, right?"

Trevin continued to look up at Thomas, trembling. Thomas flashed him a quick smile, then turned back to the others with an expression of righteous anger. He leaned down, gripping the end of their table with two meaty hands.

"How about we stick that flute up your ass and have fun hearing you play that way?" Thomas asked the flutist. "Or does that remind you too much of band camp?"

The musicians looked at each other frantically. They were only used to picking on people smaller than themselves, which happened rarely enough for them not to have developed any skills defending themselves against the more powerful. Thomas saved them the trouble of having to respond.

"How about you guys come up with something a little better than 'Oh shit.' "

Each one looked to the other to grow a backbone. Finally, one of the violinists turned to Thomas.

"We're . . . sorry?" he asked tentatively.

Thomas reached out one large paw and slowly grasped the violinist's face. His fingers gently but firmly buried themselves in the soft flesh of the boy's cheeks.

"What're you saying that to me for?" He rotated the violinist's face toward Trevin.

"I'm sorry," he squeaked out, lisping slightly because Thomas's grasp had mushed his lips together.

The other musicians quickly turned to Trevin and also offered their apologies.

"Luther would be proud," Thomas said. Satisfied, he stepped back and let the music school bullies leave, an act performed in comically fumbling fashion.

Trevin's chest heaved, as if he was breathing for the first time since the incident began. Thomas signaled for the waitress to bring his salad to the table, and he slid into the booth across from Trevin.

"You okay?" he asked, his voice returning to his normal bass lilt. Trevin just nodded. Then he blinked twice, shaking his head more slowly.

"You're bummed about the band, aren't ya?"

Trevin nodded and picked up the sandwich, which looked as forlorn as he did.

"It wasn't comin' together, Trev," Thomas told him. "Good guys and all, don't get me wrong, only cool ones around, you ask me. But . . ." Thomas gestured meaninglessly in the air as Trevin watched, chewing silently. Frustrated, unable to find words, Thomas gave up.

"We're dicks, aren't we?" Thomas said, poking at the salad that had just arrived.

"Yep," Trevin said between bites of his sandwich.

They ate their meals in silence for the next five minutes, until Thomas's cell phone rang.

Dimitri walked away from the clay tennis court on his family's estate. Bright yellow tennis balls dotted the court like a giant's Day-Glo pointillism project. He ignored the humming of the ball machine behind him—the help would switch it off and tidy up the court after he left.

Heading for the showers in the cabana, he wiped his face with a towel. The day had become so hot and humid that he had almost passed out practicing his backhand. But he didn't sweat it. He wasn't even sweating the sweat.

After last night, he felt invincible, having experienced what he only could term a miracle. However it had gone down, and he didn't look a gift horse in the mouth, Ione was no longer an issue. He had gotten a step closer to Mia.

Only three obstacles remained. Two of them were Lenore and, of course, Zander. Lenore just kept getting in the way, but she was easily dealt with if necessary. And though he was Mia's boyfriend, even Zander didn't pose a challenge. There wasn't enough to him to worry about. Mia herself was the real obstacle. She was both the opponent and the prize all along. She loved him, he was sure. In the entire school, no two people were better suited for each other. But Mia insisted on playing hard-to-get. *Because, let's face it boys, nuthin' that valuable can come easy, and both of them knew it.* So she had put Dimitri to the test and had been using Zander for the last year as a bluff. He could fold or call her on it. He'd call her up, all right. And no matter her play, he held trump. In their game, diamonds trumped hearts.

So tonight, in front of Zander and Lenore, he would present Mia a ten-thousand-dollar diamond engagement ring. It would trump Mia's desire for Zander, real or imagined, and finally, inescapably make her his own, forever.

And if that didn't work, there was Plan B.

❖   ❖   ❖

Buddy whistled to himself happily as he drove from town. When the tree-filled suburbs gave way to farmland, he could see for miles. Unfortunately, there was little to see for miles. Only intermittent clusters of farmhouses and barns broke the horizon line to the west, which was hidden by a haze of dust and humidity.

Then a cluster of shapes utterly unlike farms and houses came into view: the Fun Faire. He could just make out the Ferris wheel that towered over the tents and other, shorter structures. Closer to him on the right was a more familiar farmhouse. A quick turn and he was on the dirt road leading up to it.

The guys had been more easily swayed to re-form The Shower Tones than he had expected. Flutie had even broken into tears, apologizing for "not believing." Buddy had required no such drama, but he'd found it gratifying nonetheless. Ty had agreed to return to the fold as if he'd been doing everyone a great favor, an attitude that would probably disappear three notes into the planned rehearsal. Wes had been the big surprise, calling Buddy before Quincy had had a chance to make contact, begging him to re-form the group. He'd described going home and checking through all his teen magazines, being reminded of the success of the boy bands, even as far back as New Kids on the Block. He had convinced himself that the evolution and inevitable breakup of the current wave of bands simply meant there was now room for The Shower Tones in the universe, not that the fad itself was history.

"We could be, like, the next big thing, you know what I mean?" he had said. Buddy knew what he meant indeed.

Pulling to a stop before the farmhouse, he hopped out of the car into a cloud of dust that had billowed up. Waving it away, he called out.

"Hey, Old Man!" he yelled.

Receiving no reply, Buddy bounded up the creaky wooden stairs to the front door and hammered on it. After a moment of silence, Buddy pulled out a set of keys and unlocked the door. Normally, he didn't invade the Old Man's house, but he was starting to become concerned.

Buddy had met the old man several years ago in town. The Old Man had been impressed when Buddy had identified a tune he'd been humming, an old ragtime tune called "The Entertainer." He'd even known the name of its composer, Scott Joplin. Several months and several bottles of Jack Daniel's later, the two had struck up an unlikely friendship, but then, those were the only kind Buddy seemed to cultivate. Buddy had become a regular visitor out here. He'd sit and talk for hours with the Old Man, whose name was Joe Bragg but who insisted on simply being called the Old Man. Or if formality was required, Old Man Bragg.

Stepping in the house, Buddy listened. The house creaked comfortably around him, but there were no signs that anyone was inside. He searched it top to bottom, calling out the whole time, but much to his relief, the Old Man appeared to be out. Lately, Buddy had worried about the Old Man living so far from town alone. He'd only voiced his fears once, and the Old Man had railed at him as if Buddy'd showed him profound disrespect. Since then, Buddy had kept his mouth shut, but he'd made his visits more frequent.

Stepping back out on the porch, he realized the Old Man's junker was gone. So that settled it. He wasn't home. Must have been gone for a while, too, since he'd been calling for several hours to warn him he was bringing guests for the first time. After being banned from the Music Building, the best place to rehearse, Buddy had realized, was the Old Man's barn.

The Shower Tones were due within the hour, and the Old Man didn't like surprises, and strangers even less. But Buddy had faith that even if the Old Man discovered he'd been invaded by a fledgling boy band, he wouldn't interrupt their rehearsal. Afterwards, Buddy'd get an earful, but he was used to that. Besides, to play it safe, Buddy had brought an extra fifth of Jack Daniel's, the universal diplomat. Jack always smoothed things over.

Professor Ajit Waman unlocked his apartment, checking to make sure halls around him were empty before he opened the door. He could hear only the distant sound of a radio on an NPR station.

Once inside, he locked the door behind him, using both dead bolts and the doorknob lock. Hanging his keys on the hook near the door, he flicked a switch on the wall and the hall light went on. Its fluorescent glow revealed the shattered desk to his left and his doppelganger to his right.

Wrapped in foam packing materials, bound with plastic strips and gagged with bubblewrap lay a second Professor Waman. He lay on the floor, only his head visible, looking like a butterfly emerging from a snow-white cocoon. Bound as he was, however, this Waman wasn't going anywhere. He struggled and squinted when the unbound Waman switched on the light.

"I did not mean to wake you," said the free Waman. "Are you comfortable?"

Though not gagged, the second Waman didn't attempt to speak.

Waman began to circle the cocooned figure.

"Can you imagine?" he asked. "Something called the Fun Faire has arrived in Stratford. And an emissary visited my class today."

As he walked, his footsteps became heavier and heavier.

"How thoughtful to invite my class to the Fun Faire." His feet transformed into massive cloven hooves.

Waman laughed, his voice harsh and gravelly. The change traveled up Waman's body and arms, the muscles bulging out and hair sprouting along the way.

"Given recent events," he growled, "it will be safer to have all the students in one place, don't you think?"

Only Waman's head remained human.

"The question is, safer for whom?"

Waman started laughing, but he wasn't Waman anymore. Horns burst from his forehead, the canines in his mouth extending into fangs. His head nearly touched the ceiling.

"How do I look?" he asked with a wicked smile. The figure on the ground struggled, which only made the monster laugh.

The horned creature's form shifted once more. Orange fire burned from his eyes and hands. Soon, flickering light outlined his form. The creature collapsed into itself, forming an orange fireball that floated in place for a moment before rocketing through the window, leaving the Waman struggling helplessly against his plastic cocoon.

13

Dozens of tents clung to the western perimeter of the Fun Faire like abalone. Most were simply ragged tarpaulins roughly thrown over wooden poles, barely qualifying as tents. These clustered around a much larger, sturdier tent that adjoined the carnival itself. This tent was made of thick canvas colored the brownish red of old dried blood.

Within this tent, flickering lamps cast a dim light on a discordant gathering. Distorted shadows danced against the tent walls. These, however, were no less distorted than the figures that cast them. A man in a brightly colored housecoat, with an unnaturally tapered head, squeaked unintelligently and turned toward a hairy figure next to him. This creature whimpered quietly through his fangs in reply. Other misshapen forms could be made out: a young blonde woman with a human torso and a snake's body and a small but powerfully built man with bright red lobster claws instead of hands or feet. The further away from the light, the more monstrous and misshapen the forms became. At the center of the tent, and the strange creatures' attention, an imposing couple was in the midst of an argument.

The woman's skin was covered in reptilian scales. A spiny fin like a collar flared at her neck, flexing in her anger. The color of her scales shifted from blue to green to red and continued to oscillate.

She directed her anger at a man with smooth skin the pale color of a luna moth's wings. Long, straight white hair framed his elfin face, which rose above a powerful torso, where his body ended abruptly. He perched on a velvet-covered stool in order to see eye-to-eye with the lizard woman.

"I hate thisss placccce!!" hissed the woman. "Why have you brought ussss here, Brion?"

"Iguanita, my love." He reached out to calm her, but she stepped away, her colors and her neckfin flaring. "I have a little business to attend to before our celebration. *Our* celebration."

"Alwayssss bussssinessss," she spat. "Always meddling. You have become even more ssssecretive of late. What are you up to? Warn me now how you will ruin our anniversary!"

"Now, now," Brion laughed gently. "I am merely preparing a little tribute to you, my sweet. An offering. You will not be displeased."

"I am already displeased, Brion! If you plan a lavish celebration, why could it not be in a more lavish locale, instead of this arid wasteland?"

She spun suddenly and pointed a scaly finger into the crowd. A ripple of uneasiness went through the room, the creatures murmuring and whimpering and gibbering.

"And what about her?!"

A woman in a dark business suit, wearing sunglasses, stepped from among the crowd. For the first time, her bright smile dimmed.

"It is one thing to take her. We *take* what we need. But to send her back out?! She could have been recognized!"

"You know full well, dear," Brion answered calmly, "one cannot recognize what one has never seen."

"No matter," said Iguanita. "She will not leave here, not again."

The woman trembled at Iguanita's rage.

"You have nothing to fear," Brion assured her. "Think not that my wife is ungracious. She is merely nervous with anticipation, as we all are."

The woman turned a hesitant glance toward Iguanita, who sighed and allowed her colors to settle into a dark green. Forcing a terse smile, she bowed, acknowledging the human woman's efforts.

The human's relief was instantaneous. "Thank you, my lady," she said, bowing. She then turned to Brion and bowed again. "And thank you, sire."

"Not at all, child," said Brion. "We should be thanking you. Because of you, tonight we will all be together, celebrating, feasting and being entertained." He placed a hand upon her head as a blessing.

"Go now, dear Audra," he said. "Go with the others, and prepare."

"Yes, sire," she said and disappeared toward the back of the tent.

"As for the rest of you." Brion's voice thundered in the tent. All noises ceased instantly. "We have much to prepare for. I, Brion, your king, and Iguanita, your queen and my fair wife, appreciate your continuing allegiance and obedience. This has never been more true than tonight, given what we face, what we will do. What we *must* do."

The tent had fallen silent, with only the gentle sputtering of the lamps in the background.

Brion reached a hand out to Iguanita, who took it stiffly. Clearly she remained angry, but this was the time for a show of royal unity. He looked tenderly into Iguanita's eyes. She tilted her head in a formal, regal manner, but her eyes were throwing daggers. Brion, still unfazed, shot her an impish wink and turned back to their subjects.

"So go about your tasks," he commanded. "Should you need more 'volunteers' from town, you are given leave to collect them. Now go!"

Given permission to leave, the crowd broke up. Some shuffled or rolled onto the carnival grounds. Others slithered, stomped or hopped toward the tent village. Others transformed into balls of orange light and flew like ghosts through the tent walls and into the sky. As the tent cleared, Brion and Iguanita remained together, stiffly holding hands and nodding royally to acknowledge passing subjects.

A woman with leathery skin and a tooth-edged snout waited in a far corner with a young man whose skin was a series of armored plates.

"What are you not telling me, Brion?" Iguanita demanded, quickly seizing her husband by the shoulders and bringing him close to her face.

"Can you not allow me to prepare a surprise for you, my sweet?" Brion said dryly. "It makes the surprise so much more a surprise."

"It ssseemsss every time you sssurprissse me, Brion, I end up making an assssss of mysssself!"

Iguanita set him back upon his stool roughly. Brion had to steady himself to keep from falling off.

"You never did get over that," Brion said, shaking his head. "Really, dear, it's been several centuries. Let it go."

Her colors were cycling again. He lifted a finger and stroked her cheek gently.

"Iguanita," he cooed. "My Titania."

And instantly knew he had made a mistake.

"I'm *not!*" Iguanita cried and turned away, nearly shoving him off his stool. "Titania wasssss beautiful, queen of the fairiessss."

"You are still beautiful to me. You are still my queen."

She began to sob then.

"Silence! I am no longer Titania. Just asss you are no longer Oberon." Her body slowly cycled shades of blue. "I'm a hideousssss creature, and you, well, you may be only half a man, but at leasssst you resemble a man."

Brion leaped to the floor and padded over to Iguanita on his hands. Resting his torso on the ground, he wrapped one arm around her legs, nuzzling her thigh.

"You look like my wife and my queen," he told her. "And tonight, we will joyfully celebrate the anniversary of our wedding with our friends and our family."

She gazed down at him. Her bright eyes seemed to shine against the indigo blue of her skin. With a regretful smile, she reached down and touched his arm. And firmly pulled him away from her.

"Perhapssss . . . ," she said sadly. And left the tent.

When she was gone, Brion sighed his disappointment. Hopefully, she would appreciate his actions by the end of the evening. That would depend upon her remaining until this evening. It had always been hard to tell with her. She made mercurial seem serene. At least for now she was out of his hair and he could carry on. He turned to the pair that had been hovering in the shadows.

DAVID BERGANTINO   119

"Gator Girl! Armadillo Boy!"

"Yes, sire," they said together, standing at attention.

"Have you begun to prepare them?" he asked.

"According to custom," said Gator Girl.

"They will be ready in plenty of time for the banquet," said Armadillo Boy.

"Excellent!" he said, clapping his hands. "Then take me to them. Take me to the bodies."

Iguanita walked slowly through the Midway. Nearby, several of her kind in their energy forms bobbed and weaved among empty stalls, leaving showers of orange sparks that glittered as brightly in the afternoon sun as they did in the darkest of nights. Banners appeared in the wake of the fading sparks, as did stuffed animals and carnival games.

Lost in thought, Iguanita passed through, heedless of the activity. Like Brion, she had pressing matters on her mind.

Soon she approached a small building tucked on the very back of the site. Devoid of right angles, it resembled a disproportionately long and wide toolshed with a low roof. The curtain at the entrance drew aside as she neared, and a half-man, half-woman emerged from it. Upon seeing her, he bowed and curtsied, the luxurious red hair on the right side of her head bouncing with the motion. His left sleeve was rolled up to reveal a well-developed biceps coated with dust and sweat.

"The Mirror Maze is prepared," he/she said.

"Very good, Hermaphrodite. You may go."

When he/she was gone, Iguanita searched the area to make sure she was truly alone. She listened at the entrance to the Mirror Maze and heard nothing. Perfect.

Iguanita walked along the outside wall toward the back of the building. As she did, she dragged her hand against the wall. She could barely feel the rough wood against the scale-thickened skin of her hand. Knowing this simply amplified her sadness.

At last she reached the exit of the Mirror Maze. Making sure she wasn't being observed, she ducked into the back entrance, and after a short walk through a dark passageway, stood before the final mirror in the maze. It was flat and reflected her image perfectly, as she now appeared.

Her reflection disgusted her. Instead of soft, red lips, she possessed a scaly ridge that framed a thousand tiny, sharp teeth. Thin spines had likewise replaced the silky black eyelashes, which had once been long, prized as a talisman among mortals. Anyone lucky enough to discover and recognize The Eyelash of Titania was treated to a lifetime of good fortune. Her arms, once slim and graceful, now were rough and mottled. Her skin only appeared milky-white just before molting.

She raised a fist, prepared to smash the offending mirror, but the sight of her reflection's rapidly cycling colors stopped her. There was another way. And this, after all, was why she had come here. After centuries of resisting the temptation, she had finally succumbed. Was she not possessed of great power herself? Was she not queen?

She was all this. And more. And she would soon be greater still.

Opening her fist, she laid a palm on the mirror. She trembled slightly, aware of being cheated of the cool sensation she should have felt. Focusing her mind, a pulse of orange energy spread out from her hand. The entire mirror began to glow. The moment she removed her hand, the light winked out. But just as suddenly, a mirror on the wall next to the first glowed briefly. That too quickly darkened, and Iguanita, following the progression of her magic, watched as the glow appeared from around a bend. In her mind, she could see the magic traveling from mirror to mirror, back through the maze, effortlessly navigating it, until it reached the first mirror in the maze. This was the final mirror's twin, perfect and flat, reflecting exactly what stood before it.

Taking another look at her repellent reptile form, Iguanita stepped before the next mirror. It bowed out in the middle, causing her figure to widen comically. However, this was not what caused a smile to appear on Iguanita's ridged mouth.

In it, she saw that her skin had stopped color changing and had settled on a steady, translucent, milky white color.

14

The last of The Shower Tones arrived at the Old Man's farmhouse and assembled in the barn by five. Given the fact that they were due to be at the Fun Faire at 9 P.M. for a 10 P.M. performance, the rehearsal began on a panicky, uneven note. Buddy was at least able to get them started by reminding them that they were simply adding choreography to words and music they already knew quite well, and that the Fun Faire was literally a stone's throw away.

Buddy had been unworried anyway. Despite their apparent nervousness at the prospect of an impromptu performance, each member had thought to bring a shirt that fastened in the front with snaps instead of buttons. Soon, they were lined up, kicking and spinning, jumping and crotch-grabbing, and singing goodbye to their Coney Island Baby with the best come-hither leers they could muster.

✿ ✿ ✿

Lenore's winning combination finally came up. Twice. The multicolored tube top, matched with a denim skirt and wood-soled platform sandals, seemed perfect. Five minutes before Zander was to pick her up, however, it seemed like a horrible mistake. In a panic, she replaced the denim skirt with a flowered peasant skirt and the tube top *(What was I thinking?)* with a simple white blouse. She finished the ensemble with thigh-high cowboy boots. She pulled them on just as the buzzer sounded, announcing Zander's arrival.

"Be right down," she shouted into the yellowed plastic box by her front door, buzzing Zander in. Grabbing Rolf off the counter, she shot out the door. On the way down the steps, she caught her reflection in the window on the landing.

"What was I thinking?" she said out loud, suddenly feeling ridiculous. She started to turn, but a voice at the bottom of the steps stopped her.

"Hey Lenore."

Zander had seen her. She couldn't change now. Steadying herself, she descended to meet him.

"Wow," he said when she was halfway down the stairs.

"What?"

"You look, you know, great."

"Do I?" His sincerity was made especially doubtful by the fact that it was the first time Zander had made any comment at all about her appearance.

"Sure." He paused, as if he had something more to say. Appearing to think better of it, he said, "Ready to go?"

"Ready as I'll ever be," she answered.

Out on the curb waited Zander's trusty old Kharmann Ghia.

"I got an old stroller from a neighbor," Zander told her as they got in. "It's in the trunk."

He started the car and they drove in silence for a while, Lenore holding the Rolf on her lap.

"Hey Lenore," Zander said suddenly.

"Yeah?"

"Well . . ." He seemed about to say something, then changed his mind at the last second.

"What?" Lenore asked again, noticing distress on his face. "Are you all right, Zander?"

"Me? Sure. Yeah." He swallowed hard. "So what's up with you and Dimitri?"

Lenore's mind flashed to the previous evening, and the sight of Ione's dead body. Dimitri chasing her out of the apartment. And Ione's subsequent disappearance.

"What do you mean?" she asked. He was too nervous to notice her defensive tone.

"I mean, what do you see in him, really?"

"Zander, I don't need shit about Dimitri right now." Lenore breathed a sigh of relief. At least this was normal conversation and Zander didn't suspect the secret she and Dimitri shared.

"No, I'm not giving you shit," Zander said. "I mean it. I don't understand it, Mia doesn't understand it. He acts like a creep. So seriously, why do you like him? I don't think I've given you a chance to explain. Mia sure wouldn't want to hear it. But I do."

"Do I have to have a reason?"

He thought about that for a moment. "I guess not. But especially since he doesn't seem to like you too much, it might help. Is it just because he's good-looking? Rich? I mean, I can dig all that."

"Yeah, it's all that," she admitted. "And he's an incredible kisser."

"I don't wanna know that!" He pretended to be grossed out, making Lenore laugh.

"Well, you asked, silly," she said, punching his arm. "Seriously, I knew that he was the one for me the first time he kissed me."

"You just knew?" He wasn't buying it.

"Yeah! Can't you just know? Don't you believe you can just *know* about a person?"

"Like love at first sight?"

"Maybe not at first sight," she said, really thinking about it. "But suddenly. And absolutely. You just know who's right for you."

Zander watched her as she spoke, his smile fading with each word. He turned back to the road, choking up on the steering wheel.

"But what happens if that 'right' person doesn't feel the same way about you?" he asked.

"Try to get him or wait for him to come around," Lenore said. "You guys make fun of me, but at least I'm making an effort and not nursing a secret crush, ya know?"

"Yeah," he said quietly. "It's just that he's always seemed 'off' to me. And in any event, me and Mia think you can do better than that." He offered her a warm smile. "I *know* you can."

"That's sweet," Lenore told him. "But what can I do?"

Zander nodded his understanding, and they fell silent again until the Fun Faire came into view up ahead. He pulled off the freeway and onto the dirt road that led up to it. The parking lot—a barren field alongside a fence that separated it from a neighboring farm—was already pretty full. That meant most of the class was there. Students could be seen entering beneath the large arch. Like animals to the ark, they entered in twos, pushing strollers, wearing backpacks, each couple bringing with them a five-pound bag of flour.

As Zander parked the car, Lenore searched the dusty rows. She finally spied Dimitri's Mustang. A few spaces away sat Mia's BMW.

Once parked, she held Rolf while Zander removed the stroller from the trunk and unfolded it. She sat the "baby" inside it and strapped it in as best she could.

"I feel so silly," she said, walking beside Zander as he pushed the stroller across the rough ground.

"I think that's part of Waman's plan. He strikes me as a sadistic bastard."

"Yeah, I've noticed," Lenore said, and they headed to the carnival entrance. Mayflies frantically swarmed the proscenium lights, with only hours left in their brief, twenty-four-hour lives.

15

Around Brion, the tent village, much larger on the inside than it appeared on the outside, bustled with activity. The smells of roasting meats and savory sauces wafted from outside and seemed to collect about him. Tonight would be a glorious celebration, he thought, the best in centuries.

If my wife chooses to favor us with her presence, he thought silently, rolling his eyes to himself.

He shook his head in irritation, causing his velvet stool to wobble. The tent had been pitched over uneven ground. He was just able to steady himself as a man walked stiffly toward him from the Faire-side entrance. He looked mostly human, his naked upper torso hairy and well developed. Below the waist he wore purple tights and leather boots. It was the third eye resting square on the forehead of an otherwise flawless human face that marked him as other than human.

"The queen cannot be found, sire," said the man after his head twitched forward in a minute bow. Despite his stiffness, his voice was deep and haughty. "She was last seen near the Mirror Maze."

"Of course," Brion replied thoughtfully.

"If she has been taken, I will find her!" In a grand gesture, he reached to his mouth with both hands, withdrawing two broadswords, the hilts of which had been tucked into his cheeks. Leaping into a dramatic stance before Brion, he adopted a heroic and supple pose, brandishing the weapons before him. "I will find her and rescue her!" declared the Sword Swallower.

Brion nodded in appreciation. "That won't be necessary. She is in no danger. When she is ready, she will return of her own volition."

"Yes, sire."

Though clearly disappointed that he would mount no rescue mission, the Sword Swallower gave a grand and sweeping bow to his king. Standing erect once more, he inclined his head toward the roof of the tent and deftly reinserted the swords back down his esophagus.

"Now, is the Fun Faire in readiness to admit our special guests?" asked Brion.

"Yes, sire," answered the Sword Swallower, standing rigidly once more. "Even now, they gather at the entrance."

"Very good. And the entertainers?"

"Due soon after."

"Excellent!" Brion clapped his hands together. The stool wobbled, but he took no notice. "Then it is time!" Brion nearly shouted. "Leave me now."

Twitching his head slightly, the Sword Swallower walked slowly and stiffly away.

Brion took one deep breath, his nose filled with the tang of herbs and meat. Raising his hands into the air, he looked up, his eyes focused past the roof of the tent, into the sky, past the clouds.

Past this reality.

His outstretched hands began to blaze with crackling orange energy. The sparks floated upward, evaporating in puffs of white mist. A flame flickered in the center of each of his pupils, as if his eyes had caught fire. Soon, they too shed orange sparks of energy that leaped from his face, likewise disappearing in puffs of vapor.

Brion opened his mouth to speak. Orange lightning poured from his lips but did not alter the sound of his voice.

"Heavens blanket us!" he shouted to the sky. The energy burned from him, but Brion felt nothing but exultation. "Let no one leave!"

Waiting for Professor Waman, his students milled about just inside the entrance to the Fun Faire, wondering what to do next. Lenore had spotted Mia, standing in an overwrought, hunched and put-upon manner with Dimitri. Each held a bag of flour, neither properly equipped.

Almost dropping her "child," Mia tackled Lenore and Zander with a double hug as they approached.

"Oh, thank God you guys got here!" Releasing Lenore, she threw both arms around Zander and kissed his neck. "Baby, are *you* a sight for sore eyes!"

"Hi guys!" Dimitri said. A cat at an all-you-can-eat canary buffet wouldn't have looked more satisfied.

Mia hooked a thumb toward him, as if he were much farther away than he was.

"Dimbulb here wanted to pick me up and drive here. Like, me, trapped in a car with him. Like *that's* gonna happen."

"Look, it doesn't matter," Zander said. "We're all here now. Let's just get tonight over with."

"Amen to that!" Mia said and flung her arm around Zander.

"Flinging yourself at another woman's husband, Ms. Miller, threatens your standing in this class," Professor Waman said, suddenly materializing beside them. Mia fell away from Zander.

"You should stick with me, honey," Dimitri said, pulling her by the arm toward him. She resisted only slightly, her eyes glued on the professor.

"This is it, ladies and gentlemen," he told the class. "We're now about to embark on a real-time, real-world laboratory experiment. Enjoy your time here, if you must. Ride the rides, however it suits you. As you approach each situation, remember that for tonight, you are not carefree young adults on an evening of recreation, but a family, the responsible parents of an infant. I will be observing throughout the evening. You may or may not see me. More likely you will not. But you can guess that if you try to cheat or otherwise perform poorly, I will observe."

Lenore noticed that Professor Waman was much more animated tonight. In fact, the professor seemed downright excited. But his kind of excitement worried her. She'd seen teachers like him before, even in grade school: the academic predator, just waiting to pounce on an unsuspecting student with a failing grade.

"Now go," Waman told them in a commanding voice. Then he lowered it to a growl that everyone in the class could hear. "Enjoy yourselves."

His voice gave Lenore goose bumps. Others seemed to share the feeling, pausing a moment before beginning to lose themselves in the park. Waman just stood watching them, with a broad, dark smile on his face.

"Let's just get this show on the road," Mia said. She tugged at her black mesh sweater, which was more fashionable than functional. "Temperature sure dropped quickly."

She was right. And Lenore realized a sudden chill, not Waman's voice, had caused her goose bumps. She hadn't heard anything about it, but she figured a sudden cold front had moved in. Fog started to curl in the air around them.

"I'll warm you, Mia," Dimitri said, attempting to put his arm around her.

"Look, Dimbulb," she said, scooting out of reach. "We're going through with this so we can pass this stupid class, but keep your mitts off!"

"Okay, okay," he said. He spoke in a loud whisper to his bag of flour. "Mommy's got a headache tonight, Junior."

Mia ignored him and addressed the others. "Now let's go over to the Ferris wheel. That way, we can all sit together, our babies on our laps, like a nice pair of bloated suburban couples and pass this stupid class."

The Ferris wheel loomed ahead in the distance. On the walk over, the fog thickened to the point where they even lost track of the mammoth ride for a moment. When they could see the Ferris wheel again, Lenore had the overwhelming feeling the park had changed. From what she could see through the fog, all the rides were lit up and functioning, but something was missing.

"Where is everyone?" she asked.

"On rides, probably," Zander said. "Could be people a few feet away and we wouldn't know it. Wonder where this came from?"

"But I can't hear anyone, either," said Lenore.

"Fog tends to absorb sounds, too."

She pointed to the speakers on poles above them. Tinny music floated down to them. "We can hear that. And I think I hear calliope music in the distance. Just not voices."

Zander shrugged. He didn't have an answer for her, but he seemed unconcerned. Lenore decided to let it go.

"Anyone want some cotton candy?" Dimitri asked.

To their left stood a small white cart. Behind it, an old man beamed at them, excitedly anticipating customers. Lenore remembered her run-in with Violet Eyes. Despite the utterly innocuous appearance of the cart and the elderly vendor, the mention of cotton candy made her uneasy.

"Um, none for me," she said.

Zander shook his head. "Nah, me neither."

"What, you think I fit in these clothes by snacking on cotton candy, Dimbulb?" Mia said, hands on her slim waist.

"C'mon Mia," Dimitri said to her. "Let a guy buy you some cotton candy."

She crossed her arms, refusing to go.

"Then walk with me," he told her. She still didn't budge. "Don't be a bitch. Come get some cotton candy, okay?"

"You're not getting anywhere with sweet talk like that, sugar lips," Mia said.

Dimitri rolled his eyes and with great effort said, "Please?"

"All, right, whatever," she huffed, then turned quickly to Lenore and Zander, saying, "actually, I love cotton candy."

She kissed Zander quickly to remind Dimitri of the real score and took Dimitri's arm. The two turned toward the cotton candy vendor. All three, including the cart, vanished into the fog a moment later.

* * *

After rehearsal, Buddy directed The Shower Tones to wash up in preparation for the night's performance. As they took turns doing so, Buddy watched the cars gather in the field next to Fun Faire. At least a hundred people would be there tonight. What was he getting his friends into? Their previous performances had been well planned and poorly attended. Though their rehearsal had gone well, even he wasn't prepared for the number of people that appeared to be streaming into the park. The others would be mortified.

He wondered briefly if this was an elaborate joke, a plan spawned at the Music School to humiliate them all. For the first time, he considered calling it off.

The Old Man had failed to return, which also caused Buddy concern. He'd tried to call the police, but the phones were dead. And out here in the middle of nowhere, cell phones were less useful than paperweights. The fog that had materialized from north of the Fun Faire and rolled steadily toward it wasn't helping reception either, he bet. He thought of the Old Man again. Even if he was all right, Buddy didn't like the idea of him driving in fog that thick.

A few minutes later, The Shower Tones were ready. Or, as Quincy put it, as ready as could be expected under the circumstances. Buddy couldn't worry about them or the Old Man any longer. He was "on." Time to be a leader.

Piling into two cars, they drove the short distance to the Fun Faire. They were all nervous. Trevin could only speak in monosyllables, if he could muster the courage to make any noise whatsoever. Even the gregarious Thomas kept his Vandross-isms to a minimum during the drive. Buddy thought Uni seemed relaxed, but he realized the exchange student had gone almost as catatonic as Trevin.

By the time they had reached the parking lot, fog had engulfed the Fun Faire like a giant white octopus. It seemed content to rest among the rides and the tents, and not move on into town.

Walking across the dusty lot toward the carnival's entrance, no one spoke. Anticipation and desperation were running a neck-and-neck race. Buddy felt like they were gunslingers in an old Western, about to walk into a showdown. At least in the Westerns, they only had guns. And guns had the decency to kill. Here, they would face an audience with the power of ridicule. And one lived after suffering ridicule for quite some time.

Before they passed under the brightly lit arch, Buddy paused with the group.

"Group hi-five!" he announced and held up his hand.

They all slapped hands for luck.

"We are good to go!" Buddy announced. Adjusting his collar, he led them with a swagger under the arch and into the carnival.

To their astonishment, the Fun Faire was utterly deserted.

16

Dimitri practically dragged Mia toward the cotton candy vendor.

"Whoa, Dimbulb!" she ordered, pulling away. "You're not a reindeer and I'm certainly not a sleigh. Bring me the cotton candy. I'm done." Then she peered back through the fog. "Hey, where'd the other guys go?"

Dimitri looked back. "Probably went ahead to the Ferris wheel. We'll meet them there. Just chill with me for a bit."

"If you can actually chill, then fine."

"Look Mia," he said suddenly. "I like you. No one else is worth your time. Cut the act and get with me, okay?"

The intense look in Dimitri's eyes would almost have been frightening if Mia hadn't found him so ridiculous.

"Puh. *Leaze!*" she said, snorting with laughter so hard and suddenly that the contents of her sinuses threatened to empty onto her hand. "You and Lenore are a better match than I thought. You're both psycho-stalker people!"

She shook with laughter again, while Dimitri just stood quietly and watched. His look of anger and disappointment finally robbed the situation of humor.

"Let's just get some cotton candy," he said with barely controlled rage.

The two approached the old cotton candy vendor, who greeted them with a broad smile.

"Howdy, young'uns! You kids enjoying the Fun Faire?"

"Not really," Mia told the old man.

"Well, we got the best cotton candy in the world here," the vendor chirped, ignoring or unaware of what had passed between them, even though it had happened only a few feet in front of him. He leaned in and whispered, "Secret recipe passed down for centuries! And it's free tonight!"

"Here—hold onto Junior," Dimitri said, roughly thrusting his bag of flour at Mia, who took it only to keep it from falling. She didn't want it to break and get flour on her shoes.

"One please," Dimitri asked.

"Comin' right up, young fella!" the vendor said. He immediately plunged a white paper cone into the tumbler. As the vendor collected the pink, sugary wisps, Dimitri fished around in his pocket. Mia thought it was for change, even though the man had said the treat was free.

"Maybe you'll take me seriously now," Dimitri said, withdrawing a small black velvet box.

"What's that?" she asked, her eyes immediately narrowing in suspicion.

In answer, he flipped open the box, revealing a diamond large enough to make her gasp. Even in the fog-dimmed light, the rock glittered.

"What's that?" she said again in a half-whisper.

"A token of my feelings for you," Dimitri said.

His eyes were fixed upon her. But she could only see the diamond. Her hold on her bags of flour slackened, but she didn't notice that, or that her jaw had slackened as well.

"Now that's worth extra credit!"

Professor Waman appeared next to the cotton candy vendor, breaking the ring's spell.

"Would you please stop that?" Mia squeaked, breathless.

Typically, he ignored her, turning instead to the vendor.

"Here, allow me," he told the old man and reached for the cone. The vendor's bright smile faded instantly.

"I shouldn't—," he began weakly, but Waman interrupted him.

"Please," he said, but it sounded to Mia more like an

order or a threat. The vendor allowed Waman to finish preparing the cotton candy.

Mia thought she saw an orange flash from Professor Waman's hand shoot down the length of the cone and into the cotton candy drum. But it disappeared so quickly that she thought it could have been a trick of the light, a ghost from the glitter of the diamond Dimitri had presented to her.

"That's what I like to see," Waman said, swirling the cotton candy. "Well done, Mr. Carlton. You both pass the assignment. Your children are unharmed, and you've even gone the extra mile and proposed."

"Well, I'm not going to—"

"You've passed the assignment, Ms. Miller," Waman said, interrupting her. "Let's keep it at that, shall we?"

Mia clammed up.

"I've been watching you two, you four, actually. A very interesting dynamic. You, Mr. Carlton, are particularly fascinating, how you catalyze the people around you. The reactions you evoke. For the most part, you are a very selfish group, I must say. You're a group of *me-me-mes*."

Waman drew his lips back in a snake-grin at Mia. She retreated from his gaze and drew close to Dimitri. As he spoke, Waman lifted the cone from the drum. Instead of being pink, the cotton candy was purple, a dim black-light glow at its core.

"Of course you take that personally, Ms. Miller, but I am describing all of you. But your *me*-ness is ultimately about Mr. Carlton, isn't it? Lenore, poor girl, is in love with him. You, Ms. Miller, shy away from Mr. Carlton because in most ways, he truly is your perfect match, and that just freaks you out. Zander holds on to you only to give himself the illusion that he can compete with Mr. Carlton."

He offered the purple cotton candy to Dimitri, who made no move to take it.

"Let's make this more interesting, shall we, Mr. Carlton?" he said. "Take it."

"What do you mean?" asked Dimitri, slowly taking the cotton candy from the professor.

"Extra credit," Waman said.

"What do we need to do?" Dimitri asked. He held the cone away from his body, as if Waman had handed him a grenade.

Professor Waman smiled at him. "You'll figure it out. Now, be a gentleman and offer your wife some cotton candy."

Lenore was frantic. They called out and searched, but they couldn't even find the cotton candy vendor, let alone their friends. Zander's calm wasn't helping any, either.

"This is impossible," she said. "They were right here!"

"The fog's really thick," Zander said. "They could have walked right past us a zillion times."

"Maybe," she said. "But it's like the whole area changed. There was nothing near the cart. There's a tent here, now."

"Yeah, I know." Zander didn't know what to make of it either. "Come on, let's head to the Ferris wheel. I could use a couple minutes with you anyway. We need to talk."

He grabbed her hand, and she looked down at it.

"So we don't get separated," he said, a little embarrassed. But he didn't let go. "Come on."

"What's up?" she asked, his awkwardness growing

"Well, you know earlier, I was asking you about Dimitri?" Zander said. "And why you're so into him, and what to do about someone you like who isn't into you?"

"Yeeaahhh . . . ," she said, drawing out the word, suddenly feeling as awkward as him.

"Well, I've been wrong about you all this time," he said, gathering momentum. "I admire that you've been going for it, like you said."

He paused, but Lenore just waited for him to spit it out.

"So, um, this is me going for it." He flashed her a sheepish grin and kissed her on the mouth.

"Oh, God!" cried Lenore, recoiling from Zander. He reached out to her, but she wouldn't let him touch her.

"Look, Lenore," he cried, pleading. "It's you. I'm all about you."

"But Zander, we're friends. Just friends. This will ruin everything!" She didn't know what to say. "What about Mia?"

DAVID BERGANTINO143

"This isn't about Mia," he said.

"Everything's about Mia," Lenore told him. "And you're dating her. One way or another, this has got to be about her. You can't deny that."

"So I'll deal with that."

"I'll have to deal with it, too, you. She is my best friend."

"Then we'll do it together." He bowed his head. "I've always felt strongly about you. It's just taken me a while to pull free of Mia's gravitational pull."

He went in for another kiss. "I love you, Lenore."

"NO!" she screamed and pushed him away. Zander stumbled back and collapsed to his knees. He looked to the ground. His hair covered his face, but he appeared to be crying quietly. Her terror and shock maxed out.

"Look, I'm sorry," she said softly, putting her hand on his shoulder.

He looked up. She brushed his hair aside; sure enough, tears streaked his face. She offered him a tissue.

"Hey, you never saw me crying over Dimitri, did ya?" she asked, trying to lighten things up as he wiped his eyes.

"That doesn't mean you don't cry over him," he said.

"True," she admitted. "But let's talk about this later."

"Will your feelings change later?" His voice had a bitter edge to it.

She took a deep breath. "Honestly, no, I bet they won't. But we're friends. Like you said, we can talk about this. Just . . . right now we should find Mia and Dimitri."

He fell silent. She gave him a moment before pulling him from his knees.

"Come on," she said. Holding his hand, she tugged him toward the Ferris wheel. She thought it seemed further away than it had been a moment ago.

In the distance, someone screamed. The fog made it hard to tell which direction the sound had come from.

"At least someone's having fun here," Zander said dully.

When they arrived at the Ferris wheel, it was turning, but the cars seemed to be empty. The operator stood before a set of controls, his back to them.

"Excuse me," Lenore called out to him. "Have you seen . . ." Her voice trailed off when the man turned to face her.

"What can I do for you, young lady?" asked the man brightly.

Though clearly in his forties, he oozed the virility of a twenty-year-old. A thick, well-groomed beard and mane of hair attested to his undiminished masculinity and animal attractiveness. The blankly happy look in his eyes indicated that the mind behind them was not bustling with activity. But it was the man's eyes themselves that concerned Lenore.

They were a bright, crystal-clear violet.

❖   ❖   ❖

Perry and his "wife," Melanie, walked through the Midway. Not knowing what to say to her, he passed their time stammering out a description of his last few months of adventures on the Internet game called EverQuest. It was the only thing the pimply freshman could think to say to her. It was the only way he could get his tongue moving in her presence, even if he then had trouble stopping it. She terrified him. Any why not? Melanie was built with enough curves to give him whiplash if he looked at her too long.

After he had related the glorious conclusion to a particularly bloody quest and received a sullen glare in return, he decided to change tacks. He squeaked out that maybe the Midway would be fun; he was quite a gamer. Perhaps a stuffed animal would elicit a more cheerful response than, "Uh, right." Certainly offering to carry their flour child, which he had named Maxis Balloozog after his EverQuest character, had not impressed her.

"What do you think?" he asked. They had passed by the Balloon Races, Ring-the-Bottleneck, Free Throw, and Whack-a-Mole. Melanie had sniffed at each one.

"Where'd everyone go?" she asked. The Midway was deserted, except for one old man who seemed to be running all the games on his own.

"Well, judging by the screams," he answered, trying very hard not to stare at her breasts and finding himself fixated on her plump lips instead, "everyone's either in the fun house or on one of the rides."

Melanie frowned. She had heard the screams, too. "Feels more like Halloween than summer."

Perry felt the same unease, but he was chalking it up to the effect of Melanie's pheromones on his inexperienced libido.

"How about Flippy Frogs?" he said, trying to change the subject and focus his mind. "I'm great at this."

"Uh, right," she said unenthusiastically. She made a face at the stuffed animals hanging above them. "They look like they have fleas."

"I'm sure they're fine. It's just the fog and the lighting." His voice only cracked once that time. He waved at the game attendant, who currently stood fiddling with some tubing over at the Balloon Races. The man waved back and attached the tubing to a water gun. He walked toward them, wiping his hands on his vest and pausing once as another distant scream floated in on the fog.

"Free play tonight," the man said cheerfully.

"You ever get confused for a pirate?" Perry asked him, noticing a patch over one of the attendant's eyes.

The man's good eye clouded over a second, and his hand reached up to touch the patch. For a moment, Perry thought he had blundered big time, when he'd just been trying to make a joke. Then the man seemed to return, and he smiled brightly.

"Arrr, young man!" he said, poorly imitating a pirate. "That I be. Now ya get three tries, although since tonight's a special night, you can have all the tries you want."

He pointed to the table behind him. Metal lily pads navigated random paths over unseen grooves cut into the surface. The man held up a foam rubber frog and flopped it onto the table like a dead fish.

"Load this here frog on the frog-a-pult—we're not flinging cats in this game, just frogs, so it's a frog-a-pult—and launch your frog at the lily pads. Land two in a row on a lily pad, you get a medium prize."

He bopped a scruffy-looking, unidentifiable creature hanging from the roof of the booth. A domino effect soon set the multitude of stuffed animals dancing above them.

"Three in a row, and you get one of the big prizes!" the pirate announced. He indicated stuffed animals the size of full-grown sheepdogs hanging behind him. As an example, the pirate loaded the rubber frog onto the frog-a-pult and, without even looking, launched it into the air. It flipped and twisted—and landed squarely on a metal lily pad.

"See?" said the man. "Easy as pie!"

"Okay, I'll start with six," Perry told him. As the pirate heaved a squirmy pile of rubber frogs onto the counter, Perry unstrapped the harness that held Maxis Balloozog to his chest.

"Here, hold little Maxis," he said, handing the contraption over to Melanie. She took it as if he were handing her a dirty diaper.

"Uh, right," she said and set it on the counter beside her. Immediately bored, she leaned on her elbows next to it.

"Okay, fire one!" Perry called out and launched the first frog into the air. "Go, go, go!" he cried, willing it to land on a lily pad.

With a bounce, the frog settled on a lily pad, its limbs draped over the edges of the metal flower welded onto it.

"Woo-hoo!" he cried.

Melanie reacted with all the enthusiasm of a lobotomy patient.

"Good shot, lad!" said the pirate.

"Okay, fire two!"

Another frog flopped into the air. This made a one-point landing on a lily pad.

This time, Melanie showed some real spirit by shifting slightly so that her chin rested more comfortably on her elbow. In doing so, she knocked over Maxis Balloozog; it fell over onto a nearby frog-a-pult, but she was too intent on being bored with Perry to notice anything else.

"All right, here comes lucky number three!" The strap to the baby harness had crept into Perry's way, so he pushed it aside before his final shot. Not paying attention, he bumped her arm in the process.

"Hey!" Melanie cried out before she lost her balance, slamming her hand on the counter to stop herself from falling. Instead of the counter, her hand came down on the frog-a-pult upon which Maxis had fallen. Melaine lifted her hand to find more solid purchase, and the frog-a-pult sprang up, launching the bag of flour.

All of them—even Melanie—watched as the bag of flour tumbled over and over, sailing toward the fake pond. Maxis Balloozog landed dead center on a lily pad. The sharp edges of the metal flowers tore into the bag, and it exploded in a cloud of white.

"Um, nice shot," Perry said nervously. Turning to the pirate, he asked, "Does that count as our third?"

He had turned to address the attendant, but the man had vanished.

"How negligent," said Professor Waman, who suddenly appeared behind them.

Melanie groaned at the sight of him but said, "My bad. I wasn't paying attention."

"I noticed," said Waman. An instant later, orange light burst from his body. In his place stood a giant horned creature, with claws and hooves and fangs.

Perry and Melanie grabbed each other instinctively at the horrifying sight. Both screamed as the creature scooped up a rubber frog in each claw. To Perry's secret shame, he realized that his scream was considerably higher-pitched than hers. On the other hand, they were holding each other.

In the next moment, the beast shoved the dense rubber frogs down their throats at the same time.

Perry dropped to his knees. He collapsed against Melanie, who clawed at her own throat. The last thing Perry saw, framed by the two rubber frog's legs that protruded from his own mouth, was the creature that had been Professor Waman, laughing as they died.

17

"Are you sure you got this right?" Quincy whispered to Buddy. "This place seems empty."

The rest of The Shower Tones stood a few feet away, exchanging mutinous glances, Buddy noticed. But the only sign indicating the Fun Faire was open were the lights and, in the distance, the slow turning of the Ferris wheel. Buddy closed his eyes. Then he heard it.

"Listen."

This caught the entire group's attention. Almost in unison, the other seven members tilted their heads in the direction of the Ferris wheel.

Screaming.

"See?" Buddy said. "They're just elsewhere."

"Um, Buddy?" asked Trevin. "I-I-thought I saw M-M-monarch bumper stickers on some of the cars. This isn't a g-group from the university, is it?"

"It'll be cool. Trust me." Thomas had told Buddy of the run-in at the diner earlier that day.

The fog parted, and a figure emerged. Despite the time and weather, she wore sunglasses.

"Mr. Bragg!" said the woman, forcefully extending her hand.

They shook, and Buddy thought he heard the crunching of bones in his hand. He sure could feel them.

"I am sorry to keep you boys waiting," she said to the rest of the group. "So many guests, so many preparations, so much to do."

"No prob," he told her, rubbing his hand. But that didn't stop him from flashing her a smile to rival her own. "We're ready. Just tell us where to go and what to do."

"Please come with me," she said, beckoning them forward like they were a busload of foreign-speaking tourists.

"So what's the scoop, Ms? . . ."

"The scoop, Mr. Bragg, is that I will introduce you to this evening's celebrants. How's that?"

"Sounds peachy," he said. "May I ask your name?"

"Oh yes, how rude of me." She momentarily seemed flustered. "I'm thinking of so many other people right now, I forget myself. My name is Audra."

"Pleased to meet ya, Audra." Buddy gave her a small wave. He didn't want his hand crushed again. "You know, you look familiar."

"Very happy to meet you, too, Mr. Bragg," she said.

And to Buddy, she indeed was happy to meet him. A Zoloft kind of happy, he noted.

"I'm originally from Stratford. But that seems like so long ago."

With that, she stopped short so suddenly that the rest of the group nearly walked into her.

"Here we are!"

They had come upon a long, low tent of ragged gray canvas. Garish pictures were painted on the wall of the tent. Simple line drawings, they were drawn in an old-time style, like those in a children's coloring book.

"This is the prize attraction at the Perpetuals' Fun Faire," Audra told them. "The Cavalcade of Oddities! Let me give you some background on your audience before we meet them."

"You mean the freaks!" Flutie said. He slapped Trevin on the back. "Dude, we're gonna perform for the freaks."

"Bigger losers than us," Ty snickered. "Just the kind of boost we need."

"Gentlemen!" Audra said, her voice suddenly harsh and clipped. "We don't use the word 'freaks' here at the Fun Faire. Oddities, yes, because each one is a unique creation of nature. But never freaks. Is that understood?"

Buddy could feel her eyes burning even through her sunglasses. So could the rest of the group; Trevin hid behind Thomas.

"It's cool, lady, we're cool," Thomas said.

Audra studied them, her mouth shrunk to a wrinkled beak on her face. Buddy was certain her sunglasses were about to melt, when suddenly she was all sunshine and honey again.

"Great!" she cried, then leaned in chummily. "That's always such an awkward moment, but you know, everyone and everything deserves respect, don't you agree, boys?"

At first, they didn't know what to say. Then her eyebrows disappeared below the top of her frames, though her smile shined brightly as ever. Understanding that they were being judged, The Shower Tones enthusiastically and noisily agreed with her.

"Super! I know you boys are uncomfortable, but they're just like you and me," she said. "Just some of them have different bits and pieces. This should make you more comfortable, so just come with me."

Uni bowed before her. "We thank you for your time."

Pleased, Audra bowed back. "Why, aren't you the cutest? I think I might keep you for myself after the performance, you cutie!"

Embarrassed, Uni shrank back between Flutie and Quincy.

Audra led them a few feet along the tent wall and stood beside the first illustration.

"This is Hermaphrodite, the Bridegroom," Audra announced.

This illustration showed a bisected human figure. The right half was male, dressed in a tuxedo, sporting a handlebar mustache and greased-down black hair. On the left, he became a she, with flowing red hair, bright red lips and dressed in a wedding gown.

"Superficially, one thinks of this creature as half man and half woman, but here at the Cavalcade of Oddities, we present a being not half formed, but fully realized." Audra's voice cracked with emotion.

"Yeah," Wes said. "I mean, you got your yin yang right there. Most people are only one or the other." He examined the illustration a bit more and then frowned. "Still, it's gotta be lonely. I mean, even if you're perfect, you need other people. It's like you can get bored with yourself, you know what I mean?"

"Well said," Audra said, sniffling a bit. "What's your name?"

"I'm Wes Camacho. I sing baritone."

"Well, Bobby will be pleased to meet you, Wes Camacho who sings baritone. I know I am."

She led them to the next illustration, and they all crowded forward. Shyness gave way to excitement. They completely lost all apprehensions.

She sure knows how to work it, Buddy thought. He was almost jealous.

Audra now stood before the drawing of a well-proportioned naked woman. Above, she sported lush blond hair and the kind of breasts that would have made Lara Croft feel inadequate. From the waist down, however, the woman had a tail instead of legs.

"Is she a Mermaid?" Quincy asked.

"No, we haven't got one in our Cavalcade," Audra answered. "But that's not a bad idea." She ran her hand along the woman's tail, accentuating the curves with sweeps of her hand. When she reached the tip, she stopped and said, "This is Serpentina, the Snake Woman. Born in the Amazon." She leaned in to them and whispered conspiratorially. "Between you, me and the chickens, the proportions are a little exaggerated."

"Don't matter," said Thomas, smacking his lips. "Cuz there's a woman who can hold me *tight!* Luther loves a girl who can hang on for the ride!"

"Not many men appreciate Serpentina that way, Mr? . . ."

"Tinker," he said with a bow. "Thomas Tinker. You just call me Thomas."

"Thomas it is, then," she gushed. "Call me Audra."

"I can tell you why Miz Tina don't have more suitors. It's cuz most men are afraid of a strong, fine female. Like my buddy Wes here said, if she got the Yin, I got the Yang. And plenty of it!"

Audra found this highly amusing. The rest of the group rolled their eyes at their friend; however, they found him no less comical.

"Now let's move on," Audra said, bringing them to a lurid drawing of an alligator with red hair. "Of course, her hair isn't blond like this," Audra told them. "Not since the forties, I'm told."

She launched into an introduction of the Gator Girl, whose heavy armor of scales won the admiration of Quincy. Audra had succeeded in doing something even Buddy had never accomplished: she had dismantled all of the students' defenses and made them feel completely at ease. They talked without fear of the beings they would meet inside.

It had been three days since his capture and imprisonment, but soon he would be free. First, he had to get the hair out of his eyes; rolling on the floor toward the desk, the ponytail had wound around his head. Once he could see again, he rolled onto his stomach.

He wiggled and rocked, not rolling, focusing on the long splinters of wood from the shattered desk that lay beneath him. Creating a sawing motion with his body, he soon heard a "pop" as a particularly long splinter pierced one of the packing bubbles that bound him. Increasing his effort, he heard more popping and felt sharp pain near his left rib cage.

Good, he thought, moving slightly to the side, rocking even harder. The pain traveled across his chest to the left, then down. Not long after, he felt the jagged edge of broken particle board on his hand. Scooting up a bit, his hand was able to close around the splinter. It was about the size of a dagger.

Once he got a good grip on it, he rolled onto his

back and turned the splinter around. Drawing it upward and downward, he cut himself out of his Styrofoam prison as if he were filleting a fish from the inside. Soon, he had both arms free and was able to slip the plastic cords from his legs and shoulders.

For the first time in days, he stood up. He was free.

Near the door, light glinted off a cluster of metal objects on a hook. Keys. Among them, car keys.

His ponytail whipping behind him, he ran for the basement garage.

They arrived at the entrance to the Cavalcade of Oddities, right after Flutie commented that he envied the ability of the Armadillo Girl to curl into a ball and roll away from danger. Audra assured him that was a myth. And furthermore, the Human Armadillo was male.

"Well, I mean his sister then," he said, somewhat embarrassed. "It's just hard to tell from the picture."

"Honestly," Audra gushed, giving him a hug. "We just hired you boys because of your talent, you are all so delicious!"

While they all kicked the dirt in cartoon embarrassment, Audra pulled back the flap covering the entrance to the Cavalcade of Oddities and began to usher them inside.

"Let's go meet your fans-to-be, shall we?"

"Hey wait!" Quincy said after half the group had disappeared through the tent opening. "Where's Buddy?"

18

Colored lights flashed above them, creating three-dimensional shadows that floated through multihued fog. From within, screams and crazed laughter emanated. Hell's fanged, smiley face beckoned them to enter the place. Lenore's fear and confusion twisted a double helix of rising terror before the Fun Faire's Laugh-in-the-Dark.

"Calm down," Zander said. "Between the fog and the fact you're weirded out by that guy, we got turned around."

When she'd seen Violet Eyes at the Ferris wheel, Lenore had pulled Zander away, back toward the cotton candy vendor. Somehow, they had ended up at the Laugh-in-the-Dark, which was in the opposite direction.

"Let's find Mia and Dimitri and just get out of here," she said. "To hell with this assignment. Something's wrong here."

"Sure. Right," Zander answered. He had been sullen since she had rejected his declaration of love.

Looking into the sky, he pointed to the Ferris wheel in the distance. Then he angled his arm down and to the left.

"Let's head in that direction. Hopefully, we'll run into the other guys on the way. If not, we can just take off."

"We can't leave without them!"

"Sure we can," Zander told her. "You wanna leave, we leave. We don't need them for that. And they don't need us. Both of us drove."

"Look, Zander. Don't you think something strange is going on here? Those guys just disappeared. The only person we've seen since then was Violet Eyes. There's over a hundred people here and we only run into a homeless guy? What's he doing here?"

"Look, I don't know," he said. What he was really saying was he didn't care. "I'm freaked out. You're *definitely* freaked out. This assignment is bogus. I really just wanna go home and pretend tonight didn't happen. Okay?"

"But it did, Zander," she said. "We're gonna have to deal with it sooner or later."

"I choose later. Let's just get out of here."

Seeing that he was inconsolable, she agreed. If nothing else, she could use some distance between herself and Violet Eyes. She knew he hadn't met to hurt her, but just his presence creeped her out. And the emptiness she felt spooked her even more. It was like he was gone. At least his desperation had been his own.

"Fine," she said. "Let's go."

They set off toward the exit, holding hands begrudgingly. As awkward as things had become, neither wanted to lose the other in the fog. As a result, when Zander fell a moment later, he nearly took her with him. Steeling herself and holding on, she pulled him back to his feet as quickly as he had tumbled. Tie lines for a tent had suddenly appeared in their path. And stakes—one lay where his head would have landed.

"Wow. Lucky me," he said, rubbing his temple where the stake would have entered his skull.

"Where'd this tent come from?"

"I dunno. From what I remember the nearest tent was on the other side of the carnival."

Lenore looked toward the Ferris wheel again, but it was gone. Turning in place, she searched what she could see of the sky. And there it was, behind them.

"We're on the other side of the carnival," she said in a whisper.

"What are you? . . ." His voice trailed off as he also spied the Ferris wheel. He shook his head, then pointed along the side of the tent. "Let's go this way."

They rounded a corner and found themselves before an illustration of a redheaded Alligator Girl.

"That's impossible," he said. "It's like we warped across the park!"

"Now what do you think?" Lenore asked.

"I think we need a map," he answered. But she could tell that it was just bluster. He was starting to become rattled by something other than his feelings. "This way."

They plunged back into the fog.

A moment later, they were standing in front of the Flippy Funster. According to the map, it was near the front of the park, but on the other side of the Ferris wheel.

"What the hell?" Zander said.

The Flippy Funster was in operation, the cars spinning up, around and down. They could hear screaming from the cars, meaning they had found other students, at least. That was a good sign.

Standing at the controls was an elderly man, his skin deeply wrinkled and tan.

"Hey, mister?" Zander asked.

"Hiya, young man," the ride operator replied brightly, turning toward them. "What can I do for ya?"

He displayed the characteristic enthusiasm of the park's employees. But only one of his eyes twinkled. The other was covered with a patch.

Lenore took a step back, tightening her grip on Zander.

"Ow!"

She leaned in close. "It's Ass-Face," she whispered.

The man took no notice of her discomfort, smiling in cheery anticipation of how exactly he could help them.

Zander examined the guy for a moment, then just nodded for her to relax.

"Um, what's the quickest way to get out of here?"

The man cocked his head as if to think. After a few seconds, Lenore realized it was the same thing a puppy did when it didn't quite understand its master's orders.

"Hard to say," he finally answered. "Not really one to say, anyway. I just operate the ride." He pointed proudly at the Flippy Funster. Though it continued to run, the screaming had stopped. Apparently, the riders had gotten bored.

"You wanna go next?" he asked brightly.

"Uh, no thanks," Zander answered and pulled Lenore away.

"It's another homeless guy," she said when they had gotten out of earshot. "Don't you think it's weird!"

"So, carnival people hired local vagrants," he said. "Risky, but a good PR move, I'd say."

"Okay, yeah, but did they seem normal?"

"They seemed happy."

"And is that normal?" she asked. "They seemed empty. Like robots or something."

"Well, there's a good chance they're at least half-fried anyway, given their lifestyle."

Lenore grabbed his other hand and faced him.

"You were the one talking about UFOs, Zander. Maybe they've all been kidnapped, like you said, brought here and turned into UFO zombies."

He regarded her seriously for a moment, then his eyes went wide and he burst into laughter.

"You're serious, aren't you? Oh man, that's great!"

"But you said it yourself! You saw the lights! Strange things have been happening lately!"

"Yeah, but UFOs? Aliens?" His laughter finally died down, and he took a deep breath. "Look. Even the die-hard UFO nut, the kind that would wave the Welcome Space Brother sign at a potential landing event would shit his or her aluminum-foil-lined pants if aliens ever *really* showed up. Belief in aliens just distracts people from other beliefs, like religion, society, themselves. And as long as they're not going to be proved or disproved, they can go on with their so-called belief. So do I believe in UFOs? Sure, why not? Can't harm nuthin. But do I really believe that right now, aliens have been kidnapping vagrants here in Stratford in a sinister plot to tamper with their brains so they can operate carnival rides? Um, no, I don't think so."

Lenore suddenly felt stupid. Zander squeezed her hands in his.

"Look at it this way," he said gently. "You're a down-and-out, and someone cleans ya up and gives you a job, maybe money and new clothes, and responsibility. You'd be happy as a zombie, too, wouldn't you?"

"Yeah," she said. "I guess the fog's gotten into my brain."

His smile was reassuring and genuine.

"Come on," he said. "Let's go home and see what tomorrow brings."

He kissed her on the forehead and she didn't mind.

Just then, two figures emerged from the fog.

"Mia!" Lenore shouted. "We've been looking for you guys."

"Getting chummy while you were," Dimitri said. He looked down at their clasped hands, but Lenore was certain they had seen Zander kiss her through the fog.

"You cheatin' on me, sunshine?" Mia asked Zander.

"No," Lenore said, pulling away from Zander. "We just didn't want to get lost."

"No problemo," Dimitri answered. "We've gotten kinda chummy ourselves."

Mia licked the side of Dimitri's face.

"Oh, matron!" Dimitri said, looking straight at Lenore and Zander.

Through her shock, Lenore noticed the odd, distant look in their eyes, the stiff way they stood, smiling broadly the way the park employees did, but with an entirely unfriendly gleam. And she noticed that they held their free hands behind them.

"What the hell was that?" Zander demanded of Mia. He stepped forward, but Lenore held him back.

"I was hungry, sweetie," Mia said. "I can't get his taste out of my mouth. Maybe that's why."

Dimitri looked at her, and she looked back, bringing her hand to her mouth with a wide-eyed, mock "ooops!" expression.

"Well, maybe that's not the only reason I can't get his taste out of my mouth," she said. "But it shouldn't matter to you."

"Why?" Zander asked, breathing heavily, on the verge of launching himself at Mia.

"Puh. Leaze." Mia shook her head like they were stupid children. "Cuz we're gonna kill you, sillies!

At the same time, Dimitri and Mia brought out their other hands. Each held a large carving knife. Despite the gloom of the fog, the blades seemed to gleam brightly.

"It's our favorite carnival game," Dimitri said. "It's called Gut Your Buddies."

"The best part," said Mia, "is that you're both the game and the prize. After we kill you, we're gonna stuff your bodies and take them home!"

"That's not funny," Zander said. He tried to seem angry, but Lenore could hear the tremble in his voice.

"It's a laugh-riot, sweetie!" Mia said. Her eyes weren't laughing. In the darkness, they simply looked empty and evil.

"We're gonna give you a head start," Dimitri told them. "You start running and I'm gonna count to three. On three, we're coming after you." Before they could move, he started counting. "One . . . Two . . ."

On "two," he swiped at Zander with his knife.

"Zander!" Lenore cried and pulled him back. But the blood had already started flowing from a wound in his forearm.

"Do I smell smoke?" Dimitri asked with a childish giggle. "Because I do believe my pants are on fire!"

"Hurry!" Lenore shouted and pulled Zander away.

19

He'd seen her out of the corner of his eye as Audra was giving them Tip-Tip the Pinhead's short biography. He ignored the impossibility of being able to see more than even a few feet through the fog. But there she was, in the distance, surrounded by a bubble of clarity and light. Her long blond hair waved gently around her as if she were underwater. Her skin didn't just glow, it was iridescent, as if comprised of minute jewels. Despite the chill, she wore a thin, skintight miniskirt that accentuated the curves of her body with unreal precision.

In short, she was a hottie.

Her body was the shape of a tube of toothpaste being squeezed from the middle. And Buddy wanted to brush his teeth.

"Be right there, guys," he said, not waiting for a response.

While you guys are in there getting your freaks *on,* he thought, *I'll be over here getting my* own *freak on.*

Turning away from the silent entrance to the Caval-cade of Oddities, he walked toward the girl. She was looking right at him but didn't move to meet him halfway. She just stood there, waiting and glowing.

Buddy breathed on his hand, sniffed it—*no dragon breath,* he thought—and without a pause smoothed his hair so she couldn't tell what he was doing. In a few steps his saunter evolved into full-fledged mosey. Very sexy.

"Hey," he said. "What're you doing out in the mid-dle of this spooky carnival all alone?"

She didn't answer at first. Instead, she looked him up and down—then just down—and giggled.

"I'm Buddy," he said. She looked doubtfully at his hand for a moment, then reached out to shake it. "What's your name?"

"I'm B'ritnee," she said.

"Like Britney Spears?"

"I wish!" she said breathlessly. "It's B'ritnee: B-R-I-T-N-E-E, with an apostrophe after the B. Do you like it?"

"I do indeed," he said. "So are you here alone?"

"Very," she answered. She sized him up once more and her voice suddenly became a low purr. "*Very* very. Tell me, am I an attractive girl?"

She ran her hands down her sides, caressing each curve slowly down to her waist. Buddy gulped.

"B'ritnee," he said, "you got the hottest apostrophe I've ever seen. No wonder the fog burns off around you."

Satisfied, she nodded and snaked her arm around his. "Good. Then take me around the carnival. Take me on rides. Show me a good time."

She started walking, practically pulling Buddy off his feet. This one sure moved fast!

"Do you go to Globe?" Buddy asked when he regained his balance.

B'ritnee seemed to consider this question very carefully.

"I'm an exchange student, let's say," she finally answered. "What about you?"

"I'm a singer," he told her proudly.

"Oh really?!" B'ritnee squealed. "I love singers. What kind?"

"I'm the lead in a boy band."

B'ritnee yanked him to a stop, nearly dislocating his arm.

"Get out!" she shrieked. "Really?"

Buddy bobbed his head humbly. "Yes, really."

This provoked her to stroke his chest, slowly, from his neck on down.

"Mmmm . . . ," she said.

Her hand stopped at his waist, though she seemed tempted to continue. Buddy was tempted to beg her to keep going. Instead, she hugged him playfully.

"Take me to the Laugh-in-the-Dark, Buddy," B'ritnee said in a panting voice, dragging him forward. "But while we're in there, I want to do more than laugh."

Now it was Buddy's turn to stop short.

"Hey, wait. Um, you're not like, um, uh . . ."

B'ritnee didn't catch his meaning and waited impatiently for him to continue.

"This isn't gonna cost me, is it?" he finally blurted out.

"Cost you? Oh, Buddy!" she gasped, realizing what he was asking. "Cost you? Aren't you a bonbon?"

She burst out laughing and fell against him. Her body was warm and soft and made Buddy certain he was gonna pay for something. A body like that cost a man, one way or another.

Her laughing subsided abruptly, as if she'd caught herself falling or had had a depressing thought. She fell silent, continuing to hold him. He looked down and saw sadness on her face.

"It's just been a long time since I've had a whole man," she told him.

"You mean a *real* man?"

"Yeah, that too," she answered.

"I swear I've seen the merry-go-round operator in town somewhere," said John "Murph" Murphy. He was mostly talking to himself, but unfortunately he'd said it loud enough that his class-assigned wife had heard him.

Polly held up the bag of flour and made a googly face at it.

"Have you seen the nice man before, liddy biddy baby?" she asked in a slightly crazed doll voice. She paused as if to give the inanimate object time to answer, then cackled. "No, I didn't think so. No, I did not!" she told it.

Murph closed his eyes and took a deep breath. This stupid assignment was hard enough, but being paired with this nutjob really took the cake. Ironically, he had taken the class in the first place to meet chicks. Since he'd already done all the women he had met at the gym where he worked as a trainer, Human Sexuality 101 had seemed like a good place to meet young, naïve chicks. Or at least those as sexually obsessed as he was. They didn't even have to have a body to compete with his two hundred pounds of fat-free muscle. As a bonus to the prospective bedmate, a chick's gray matter didn't matter to Murph. He had more interest in the pinker parts of a woman. But he didn't care how pink Polly's parts were. She was just a wacko. Earlier, she had pretended to breast-feed their pseudo-child, pressing it to her plump chest. Never had Murph been less attracted to a chick.

"Let's just find a horse and sit down, Polly," he told her. "And will you stop talking to the fuckin' thing? It's a bag of flour for chrissakes, not a real baby!"

"Daddy's angry!" she cooed, shielding the baby in her arms. Then she lowered her voice to a whisper. A loud one. "He gets that way when he drinks."

"What the hell?!" he shouted at her. She shrank back, clutching her "baby" to her chest. He could only growl at her, "Sit back here and give it a rest. I'm gonna be up there."

He stalked forward among the painted wooden horses. He and Polly were the only ones on the merry-go-round. Which was a bummer, because he felt he'd give his right nut to talk to anyone else. Among the horses he found other creatures, including a bear, a couple of dogs and a few fantasy creatures, like a giant sea horse. Finally, he discovered a creature that matched his mood. It was some horned thing, like a ram or a goat or something. Straddling it with his legs, he looked back at Polly. Of course, she sat astride a unicorn. Head bent, she was singing softly to the bag of flour.

"God, this night can't end fast enough," he muttered to himself.

The only good thing about Polly was that she insisted on taking possession of the bag, which she insisted on calling Snuppums. That left him little to do but endure her company, but even that was verging on too much for him.

The calliope music struck up, and the ride lurched forward. He held onto the pole in front of him as the creature beneath him moved up and down.

Murph had a few moments of peace before Polly began to shout from behind him.

"Baby wants his daddy, Jonathan!" she called out. "Snuppums wants his daddy."

He tried to ignore her, but she just shouted more loudly over the music.

"Snuppums wants his daddy!"

Turning, he shouted back, "I said give it a rest, you psycho!"

"I'm going to tell Professor Waman that you're a *ba-a-a-aad* father!" she called back.

Murph leaped from the creature he was riding and stomped back toward Polly.

"That's it, gimme that!" He reached for the stupid bag of flour.

"No!" she shouted, leaning back on her mount, holding onto Snuppums with both hands.

Murph didn't even try to be delicate. Delicacy had never been one of his strong points anyway. He snatched the bag from her.

"Baby's got his daddy now!" he snarled at her. Lifting the bag over his head, he brought it down on the unicorn's horn. He pushed until the point burst through the other side, sliding Snuppums to the wooden animal's forehead. Flour poured from the two punctures like blood. Polly screamed as if it had been her he had run through.

"You murderer!" she screamed. "You killed Snuppums!"

"It's a bag of flour!" He shouted. "Flour!"

Then her hand went up to her mouth and she began to scream.

"Shut up!" he yelled. "You're gonna get us fucking arrested!"

But she didn't shut up. Instead, she scrambled backwards, nearly falling off her unicorn. Murph noticed she was no longer looking at him, but behind him. He heard a thump, and the merry-go-round lurched as if it had jumped its track.

Turning, he found himself facing the goat creature he had just been riding. Only now it was standing two feet taller than him. Looking beyond the creature, he saw that the space where he had been riding it was empty. Like it had sprouted hair and stood up.

Between the creature's inexplicable appearance and Polly's constant shrieking in the background, Murph found it too difficult to concentrate on being afraid.

While he tried to focus, the beast lifted him by the shoulders. A moment later, Murph participated in a father-son spin at the end of the unicorn's spike.

20

Sweat ran down Lenore's back despite the chilly conditions. She felt like she had a few days ago, walking to school and anticipating the sight of Dimitri, her clothes clinging to her like wet papier-mâché. Tonight, however, she felt frightened, dreading what might happen if Dimitri and Mia caught up with them. Neither she nor Zander could tell how long they had been running and hiding, trying to flee the not-so-Fun-anymore Faire. The fog had stopped time and denied them escape.

"Why can't we get *out* of here?!" she sobbed from behind a bench on the merry-go-round.

"Sssshhhh!!!" Zander said, his own chest heaving, an ashen expression on his face.

A moment ago, a woman had screamed not ten feet from where they crouched. Now no one was there. The merry-go-round was deserted. There wasn't even an attendant.

"Ghosts?" she asked. They'd been talking UFOs, so why not?

Zander just shook his head out of helplessness. He held his arm. Luckily, Lenore had pulled him back just in time, and the knife had barely touched him. But she could tell that the attack itself troubled him more than the wound.

"It's not just the sounds, it's the place. The fog." He kept his voice low. "This place isn't that big. We should be out of here by now." He swiped a hand at the mist in front of him, as if to draw back a curtain. It swirled in the wake of his hand and then mended itself. "Something is keeping us here."

"What something?"

Zander just shook his head. "Whatever it is, it did a number on Mia and Dimitri. That wasn't them."

"So we can't get out. At least the fog's keeping us apart."

"Is it?" Dimitri asked, his face suddenly appearing over the back of the bench. His smile was bright, and gleeful, and terrifying.

Mia popped up beside him, with the same malevolent expression.

"You gotta be friends with the fog, sweeties. We are!"

Lenore and Zander pushed themselves backwards, scrambling away from their former friends.

Up came the knives again, reflecting the pulsating light of the merry-go-round.

"Come on!" Zander cried and pulled himself to his feet.

Mia and Dimitri started to crawl over the back of the bench.

Zander cried out in pain as he yanked Lenore to her feet by his wounded arm. Then he practically shoved her off the merry-go-round.

She caught herself when she landed on the ground, but when she turned back she could see him falling, narrowly avoiding becoming impaled on the ride's unicorn.

The other two were almost upon him as Zander scrambled to his feet and leaped off the ride. Grabbing her hand, they ran off. Lenore looked back to see Dimitri and Mia waving with their knives from the merry-go-round, as if they were just friendly neighbors saying "Howdy" from a porch, disappearing as the ride spun them away and into the fog.

The illusion that they were in an amusement park had vanished. And Lenore finally recognized the nature of the screams they had been hearing all night. These were no shrieks of laughter and amusement. She heard them for what they were: the sounds of a slaughter.

"What's wrong?" Buddy asked as they left the Laugh-in-the-Dark. B'ritnee had become quiet and had not let him touch her as she had earlier suggested. He tried to cajole her in the best Buddy Bragg manner, pointing out how very alone they were, and how very perfect the conditions were for petting, but she had tensed up and her attention seemed to be focused elsewhere. Her face had the expression of an animal sensing a coming earthquake.

It gave her mouth a pinched quality. But that didn't mean he didn't want to kiss it.

She was ignoring him at the moment, her mind elsewhere as they strolled through the carnival, lightly holding hands. That bothered him not in the least. He was game and he *had* game, whatever *her* game.

"Pilot to tower," he said through his hands, making a radio static noise. "Permission to land."

This got her attention.

"Permission to land?" she asked. "Land what?"

"This," he said and kissed her on the lips. Nothing fancy. No tongue. Just enough to let her know he was still there.

Her expression clouded.

"The impudenssse! To defile the queen in ssssuch a manner!" She raised her hand to slap him, then froze. Buddy hoped his look of shock had stayed her hand. Because that was the oddest thing he'd ever heard fly out of the mouth of a bubbly thing. Not to mention the weird slurring of her Ss.

Suddenly, B'ritnee flushed and looked to the ground.

"Um, it was a line from a play," she said. "Sorry, you just surprised me."

Buddy saw his opening and took it.

"But I did not displease you, milady?"

She looked up sharply, searching his face to see if he was making fun of her. She decided he was not. Or that it didn't matter.

"Quite the contrary," she said, continuing the role play. "I was quite pleased."

"Then with your permission?"

Buddy went back in for seconds, pausing before he touched her. His lips hovered less than an inch before hers. He could feel her breath on his face.

"Permission granted," she said, her voice light and wispy, her eyes rolling up into her as she submitted to his kiss. And kiss her he did. Her response was ferocious. And her technique, incredible. Her tongue darted in and out of his mouth with feather-light flicks.

He pulled away and examined her face. It looked so innocent. But her tongue was obviously a repeat offender.

"Let's go in there," he said, pointing to a sign above a nearby doorway.

Like she had in the Laugh-in-the-Dark, B'ritnee tensed and pulled away.

"Let's not," she said, her mouth drawn tight once more.

"Come on. It's the Magick Mirror Maze. I bet they got those twisty mirrors, too." She wanted to pull away, but he held her hand firmly. "You know, the kind that give you a big head, or make you look fat? They're a riot. And you know what my Grams used to say?"

"No, what?"

"She used to say mirrors like that, the fun house mirrors, show how you look on the inside." Buddy laughed, but he stopped short when he saw the pained expression on B'ritnee's face.

"That depends," she said, "on which mirror you start with."

A moment before, the entrance had been only a few yards ahead. Three steps later, they found themselves standing before a tent marked Employees Only.

"I don't know how much longer I can take this," Zander panted. "Pretty soon, I'm gonna be as crazy as they are."

"This is our chance," Lenore told him. "We might be able to get some help."

"The only other people in this place are the hired help, your Stepford vagrants," he answered. "And I don't know if I want to meet the people responsible for their lobotomies."

"Look, it's right here," she told him. She ran her free hand along the edge of the opening. "And there's no fog inside, I bet."

"We gotta get out of this fog," Zander agreed.

Together, they stepped into the tent.

Immediately they knew they had made the right decision. The tent was dark, but warm. Better still, the aroma of cooking food filled the tent. It was the first bit of comfort they had experienced in hours. They couldn't even hear the screams from inside the tent.

Lenore knew just what to do. "Let's let our eyes adjust to the dark. Then let's find the kitchen, or wher- ever the food is."

"Excellent," Zander said.

"There," Lenore said, pointing to a far corner of the tent. "Over there! I think I see another door."

Moving quietly, they approached a doorway that had been hidden in the gloom. Sure enough, beyond it was a canvas passage that linked this tent with another. This, too, was unlit, but their eyes had adjusted enough to make out individual objects as shades of black.

Soon they came to a tent nearly as large as the employees' tent. An odor of overpowering pungency hit them immediately. The strong, but not unpleasant, smell seemed to be rising from a table at the center of the tent. Lenore thought she could make out the shapes of chairs pushed against the tent walls. Many of the chairs were not empty. Lenore was about to approach one when she heard Zander sniffing at the table.

"Hey, check this out," Zander said, bent over an object about the size of a bowling ball. There were dozens such objects on the table. "It's like potpourri."

Lenore joined Zander at the table, upon which rested many pots filled with water and leafy materials. The water bubbled, but she could find no heat source beneath the pots.

Now that she was used to it, the smell made her hungry. They hadn't eaten for hours. Until now, terror had spoiled her appetite.

"Let's keep going," she said. "Someone's gotta be here somewhere."

"Someone normal," added Zander hopefully.

But before they could leave the room, the passageway leading back to the Fun Faire filled with a dim, orange glow, like torchlight. Lenore started in its direction, but Zander held her back.

"But what if it's someone who can help?" she whispered.

"What if it isn't?" he pointed out. He nodded toward the floor. "Down there, come on."

Quickly, they scooted under the table.

The room brightened suddenly, but only the torches seemed to have entered the room, not the bearers. From under the table, they could see no one. The light, however, allowed them to see what filled the chairs in the room. Based on the visible boots and tennis shoes, jeans, Capri pants and skirt hems, they had found some of their classmates for the first time that night. But they weren't moving. Lenore could think of only one reason why all these people had remained so still while she and Zander had investigated the room. The reason raised a white flag in her mind, and unconsciousness started sending up black fireworks of victory.

Zander squeezed her hand, and the fireworks stopped. He was pointing toward the lights. They burned brighter, and sparks fell from the space above the table. From out of the sparks, two sets of legs materialized.

One set wore a long, brightly colored housecoat, with feet sporting fuzzy slippers. The other wore no footwear—it had three, thick toes ending in dangerous-looking talons that gouged the ground and left deep grooves in the dirt when it walked. From its ankle to its knee—and presumably higher than that—it was covered in brown fur. At first, Lenore imagined a bear had wandered into the tent.

But then it spoke.

"Let's put them here, Tip-Tip," she heard it say, its deep voice slightly muffled, as if the creature were talking through a mouth full of marbles. Or sharp teeth.

"Tip-Tip" responded with a strange series of hoots and clicks.

Both figures stood before a pair of empty chairs. The glow in the room had dimmed greatly since the two creatures had appeared. Whatever light remained flared suddenly, and sparks fell to the ground. When they evaporated, the chairs were no longer empty. Before the orange light winked out entirely, Lenore saw a set of legs appear in each chair. In one she glimpsed a thick pair of male legs clad in denim. The second pair was covered in acrylic pants.

"It will be quite a feast tonight," it said.

Tip-Tip gibbered in response, to which the hairy one replied, "It's not our job to prepare them."

More gibbering.

"He stakes 'em, we rakes 'em, and that's that," replied the hairy creature.

Even though it was unintelligible, even Lenore understood Tip-Tip's reply to mean, "Whatever."

That settled, the two mumbled just under their breath and quickly evaporated in a shower of orange sparks. Whatever they had become zipped from the room much more quickly than they had entered. As soon as the orange glow faded from the outer passageway, Lenore and Zander crawled from their hiding place.

In another minute, their eyes adjusted, and they could see. As Lenore had feared, they found the room filled with the corpses of their classmates.

Lenore stifled a scream that wouldn't have stopped save heavy sedation or death.

"Oh fuck, it's Murph!" Zander said, examining the two new arrivals. "He's been stabbed in the crotch. And that's some girl named Polly, I think. Oh geez!"

Zander doubled over, his hands on his knees. Lenore saw what he was looking at. Her skull was narrower than it should have been. Blood trickled from her eyes.

"You all right?" Lenore asked, aware of what a ridiculous question that was. Zander continued to hyperventilate.

Looking around to spare him embarrassment, Lenore found her gaze falling upon a girl sitting slumped against the wall directly across from her: Ione. Her dead eyes seemed to stare at Lenore through the darkness. Lenore could no longer suppress the scream that had been building all night.

The far end of the tent suddenly lit up. Orange light filled a passageway beyond, growing steadily brighter.

Zander clapped a hand over her mouth to silence her. Someone or something was coming.

"Come on!" Zander said, standing and pulling her back in the direction of the Fun Faire.

"We can't go out there!" she cried.

"We have to. Unfortunately, the fog seems to be the only place we can hide."

Orange sparks appeared in the far passageway.

Lenore followed Zander quickly out of the morgue tent and into the fog.

The Employees Only sign vanished in the mist behind them, and they arrived abruptly in the Midway.

Almost immediately, Lenore heard Dimitri.

"Time to play!"

Before she could turn toward his voice, she felt hands on her, lifting her.

"Heave ho!" he cried and threw her against a nearby counter. "Emphasis on the 'ho.' "

The blade flashed in his hand again. This time there was no playful flourish. He just thrust it forward into her chest.

21

They walked silently, hand in hand, through the Fun Faire. Since their kiss near the Magick Mirror Maze, B'ritnee had grown silent and introspective. Buddy could sense she wasn't exactly working up the nerve to kiss him again.

"You have a boyfriend, don't you?" he ventured.

Her shamed silence told him he was right.

"It's okay," he said. "Tell me about him."

For a few steps, she didn't say a word. Then she just started speaking, as if narrating a dream she was having.

"He's not like you at all," she said. "Let's just say he doesn't do tall, dark and handsome. He hasn't for centuries."

Buddy found her words strange, but he didn't want to interrupt her flow. He, more than most, understood the importance of "flow."

"He's not gentle like you. He's not funny like you. He's certainly not attentive. He's very busy taking care of everyone else."

His face twitched with questions, but still he didn't want to speak. B'ritnee seemed to sense his curiosity and looked up at him. She smiled, sweetly, and touched his cheek.

"You really are a doll," she said. "You see, he cares for his brothers and sisters, a great many of them. As do I. We serve as parents of a large surrogate family. It's one of our bonds. But sometimes he gets so wrapped up—and truly, they are a handful, which is especially burdensome when you use your hands for everything—I just feel . . . lonely sometimes. And sometimes I would like to be free of all that responsibility."

"I know what you mean," he said, finally feeling comfortable enough to speak. "Not a big fan of responsibility myself."

"I can sense that," she replied.

"I'll take that as a compliment. But no wonder you're such a contradiction. Having to care for a family at your age, dating a difficult guy. You're beyond your years, like an old woman trapped in a young girl's body."

"You could say that."

"Personally, I think it's a great combo," he said with a wink. "And bonus, you haven't lost your looks. Stress like that can grind a person down hard."

"Yes, exactly."

"And by the time you're thirty, you're sitting with two screaming little kids, each of you with a bottle, except yours says Jack Daniel's, because he's the only man you can rely on to be home every night. Soon, you're looking like the Creature from the Black Lagoon and your old man, he won't want ya anymore. Guys are jerks. I'm a guy and I know that. You're better off without him, B'ritnee."

"I used to roam freely with my own family," she said. Her knitted brow hinted at a conflict raging behind her eyes. "But where would I go these days? And deep down, I know he wants me. He may be cold at times, but he wants me."

"Maybe. Now. But that's because you're young and beautiful. Everyone thinks that, then old and wrinkly happens. Might as well have as much fun as you can, while you can."

B'ritnee regarded him with a curious expression.

"So tell me, Buddy Bragg. Are you wise or just cynical?"

Buddy could feel his face getting hot. She was looking into him now, not at him. He looked at his feet.

"I'm twenty-seven, still a college student and this week, I head up a boy band. You tell me."

An amused smile played on her lips, and the two continued walking in silence. Buddy became lost in his own introspection, but with some difficulty. His emotional muscles ached from disuse.

Something ahead broke the melancholy spell B'rit-nee had cast upon him.

"Hey, lemme buy you some cotton candy, okay?" he said. Without waiting for an answer, he headed for the vending cart that had come into view just ahead.

"No, I don't think that's a good—"

"Old Man?" Buddy said when he got a good look at the old cotton candy vendor. He let go of B'ritnee's hand and ran ahead. "What are you doing here?"

"Hello, son!" said the Old Man. "Some cotton candy for you and the pretty lady?" There wasn't an ounce of recognition in his eyes.

The fact that the Old Man was smiling at all immediately told Buddy something was wrong.

"It's Buddy, Old Man."

The Old Man continued to look at him cheerily.

"I'm sure you're everyone's buddy," he said. "Now how about some cotton candy?" He held up a white paper cone as if he were presenting the Holy Grail.

"You know him?" asked B'ritnee.

"He's a friend. He lives on a farm out here." Buddy thought he caught a flicker of recognition in B'ritnee's expression. And a glimmer of guilt. The Old Man, however, continued to stand by, holding up the white cone. He didn't move, as if he were a robot waiting to be activated.

"The Old Man was missing when I got to his place today," Buddy told her. Then he turned to the Old Man, who blinked twice, as if coming online. "Okay,

Old Man. You don't recognize me. But do you know
who *you* are?"

"Why, I'm a proud servant of the Perpetuals," he
said without hesitation. "I sell the finest cotton candy
from a centuries-old secret recipe!"

Using the cone, he swirled up some cotton candy.
As he did so, B'ritnee's eyes widened in shock.

"What?" asked Buddy.

"Try some!" said the Old Man, thrusting a puff of
purple cotton candy between Buddy and B'ritnee.

All fears for the Old Man, and all other thoughts,
got drowned out in the ocean roar of Buddy's sudden
desire for the cotton candy in front of him. It seemed
to pulse steadily, like a gauzy heart. He reached up to
pull a tuft of it away.

"Sssstop!" B'ritnee cried and knocked the cotton
candy out of the Old Man's hands.

Did she just hiss? Buddy wondered absently as his
eyes followed the cone's descent to the ground. He
almost dove for it. But the moment it hit the ground,
his mind suddenly cleared. The Old Man, suffering
from amnesia—could it be a stroke?—stood next to
him, and all he could think about was cotton candy?
What was up with that?

"Sssstand back," B'ritnee suddenly ordered.

"Aw look, ya dropped it," said the Old Man. "I can
make ya a new one lickety-split, though."

He reached for a new cone, but B'ritnee roared at
him.

"I ssssaid *sssstand back!*"

The Old Man stumbled away as B'ritnee laid her hands on the cart. To Buddy's amazement, her hands glowed orange, and soon the entire cart was suffused with orange light.

The rumbling of the machine's motor grew louder and rougher. The cart started shaking. The thing was going to explode.

Heedless of the energy pouring from B'ritnee, Buddy reached for her arm to pull her away. It was like grabbing an electric eel. A thousand needles ran up his arm in the moment of contact. He pulled back so hard that he fell onto his butt.

The cart began to shake more violently, hopping up and down in place. Lifting her hands, B'ritnee quickly darted behind the cart, where the Old Man continued to cower. She yanked him toward Buddy. She was no longer glowing, but some unearthly strength allowed her to pull Buddy to his feet and fling him and the Old Man away from the cart. From the ground behind B'ritnee's feet, they watched the cotton candy cart melt down.

Purple sparks flew from the drum mechanism, giving the scene the surreal appearance of a neon-violet volcano. The awning over the cart collapsed and fell to the ground. The cart's sides began to buckle outward, metal groaning, rivets creaking.

A moment before it seemed ready to explode, the sides of the cart bulged outward with a muffled pop.

Instead of exploding, the sides crumpled in, imploding in the grip of a tremendous invisible hand. A ball of purple fire shot into the sky, exploding like fireworks, the sparks dissipating quickly.

The mangled cart stopped glowing and tumbled to its side.

Buddy was stunned by what he saw, but B'ritnee gave him no time to reacquaint himself with reality.

"Get up," she ordered.

Her hands began to glow again. And Buddy Bragg knew enough to back off from that action. So did the Old Man, and the two of them shrank away from her. Her hands held before her, a globe of energy formed around them. The fog shrank back from the energy, not evaporating, but actually retreating. The field of light expanded, creating a hole utterly devoid of fog. Buddy could hear B'ritnee mumbling under her breath as she reached forward, pushing the ball away from her. The globe stretched before her, then rapidly shot forward, boring a tunnel in the dense fog. For the first time since his arrival, Buddy could see details of the carnival in the distance at ground level.

B'ritnee turned to them. Her hands were no longer glowing. But her eyes were.

"Come with me," she hissed at him. "Bring the Old Man. Your friendssss are in danger!"

With little other choice, or the mental capacity to make one, Buddy stepped into the tunnel with the Old Man in tow.

22

After stabbing her, Dimitri thrust his face into Lenore's. By his expression, he was clearly looking forward to watching her die an agonizing death, up close. Lenore looked over his shoulder, mostly to avoid his maniacal gaze, to find both Mia and Zander frozen in place. Zander's face had gone white. And the sight of Dimitri's knife buried to its hilt in Lenore's chest seemed to have put Mia's murderous rampage on Pause.

Luckily, Lenore felt no pain. She'd been worried about that. She didn't want to die painfully. A long moment later, she noticed something strange.

She wasn't dying at all.

Dimitri's face suddenly changed. He looked confused and disappointed. Together, they looked down at the knife handle that protruded from her chest. Something poured from the wound where the blade had entered, but it was not blood.

Flour.

Dimitri had stabbed Rolf, who had been resting in her chest carrier, stopping the blade before it could pierce her skin.

They looked up at each other at the same moment. Dimitri's eyes showed fear for the first time. There was good reason for that, because now, Lenore was pissed.

Before Dimitri could move, Lenore grabbed his hand, trapping the knife in the flour bag. Then she headbutted him. He reeled back, crying out and letting go of the knife, as she'd intended. Through the pain of the blow, she pulled the knife from the flour sack and threw it to the back of the stall behind her.

Mia cried out as Zander disarmed her as well.

"We're all gonna calm down," he began. "And talk about—"

He didn't get to finish before Mia leaped upon him, knocking him to the ground. She straddled him and went for his eyes. Zander grabbed her by the wrists just in time. Whatever had possessed her had made her strong. He was just barely able to keep her from clawing his eyes out.

"I don't need a knife, either," Dimitri said, suddenly in Lenore's face again. And his hands at her throat.

Lenore couldn't breathe, but she didn't even try to pry his hands off. A knee to his balls immediately loosened his grip.

"I've had about enough of you," Lenore cried.

While Dimitri stood doubled over, groaning and clutching his groin, Lenore ran to the Whack-a-Mole machine. The mallets were tethered to the machine by rotting cords. With one firm yank, the cord broke, and she returned to Dimitri. He was struggling to stand properly. In the distance, Mia and Zander continued to wrestle, rolling over and over. No immediate danger there.

Dimitri straightened up just in time to catch a blow from the Whack-a-Mole mallet on the side of the head. He staggered to the side. The mallet was padded but dense. She hadn't given him a love tap.

"I've loved you since we first kissed, and you've treated me like shit!"

Whack! She struck him with a two-handed blow that nearly knocked him off his feet.

"You won't leave my friend Mia alone, who obviously doesn't love you. I mean, get real!"

Wham! An uppercut to the chin, and he staggered backwards. A seam on the leather mallet head popped and started leaking sand.

"Now you've been trying to kill me all night?"

Whack! Whack! Whack! She pelted his body, rather than his head, with blows so she wouldn't knock him unconscious yet. She wasn't quite finished.

"If you won't love me, I'd rather you were just dead!" she screamed. Winding up like Barry Bonds, she put her entire body into a swing. When the mallet connected with Dimitri's head, the seams exploded, sending sand everywhere. Dimitri flew backward, seemed to hover horizontally for a moment, then fell to the ground and lay still.

Now she was finished.

She stood breathing heavily, shock and overwhelming satisfaction wrestling at odds within her. Still holding the wooden handle to the mallet, she stepped over Dimitri's body toward Mia and Zander. They had rolled under the Flippy Frog counter. Zander was on his back; both were strangling the life out of each other. Lenore raised the mallet, but Zander made a move. He shoved Mia upward, slamming her head against the bottom of the counter. The first blow loosened her grip on his neck. The second knocked her unconscious.

Wearily, he rolled her to the side and stood up, rubbing his throat. He looked from Dimitri to Mia, then up at Lenore.

"Are you okay?" he asked.

"Yeah," she replied dully. Her arms hung limp at her sides, but she continued to grip the handle tightly. She didn't fear Dimitri or Mia any longer, even if they did somehow come to. But she couldn't let go of the mallet. It seemed to be a part of her. And she didn't know what else would emerge from the fog.

Zander put his arms around her and held her for a moment.

"It's okay," he whispered in her ear. "It's over now."

Then he lightly kissed her ear. Then her cheek.

Then her lips. And then his tongue was in there and he was holding her even more tightly, caressing her body. Lenore shrieked and pushed him away.

"What the hell are you doing?!" she yelled.

"I don't know," he said, looking at the ground. "I just thought . . . what we've been through . . . look, I still feel the way I feel, okay?"

"Not okay," she growled. Her rage flared within her once more. Without thinking, she brought the handle up in a lightning-quick backhand and struck Zander in the temple. He dropped to the ground like a stone.

Now she was truly alone. Her friends lay strewn about the ground beneath her like discarded rag dolls. The fog continued to obscure the carnival around her. Even the screaming had stopped.

She dropped the mallet handle to the ground.

Behind her, someone applauded.

Lenore spun quickly to find Professor Waman standing there. He stopped clapping and crossed his arms.

"Very nice work, Lenore," he said. "Worthy of my own efforts. Well, at least it would be if you had actually killed your friends. Too bad you'll fail the class anyway."

"Why are you still talking about your stupid class?" she asked wearily. Surrounded by her unconscious friends, moments after almost being killed by two of them, the concerns of the Globe University campus seemed a continent away.

"I care about the class," Waman told her. "And you should have, too. Looks like only four in the entire hundred or so of you will pass this class. You should have taken care of your child."

It took a moment for his words to sink in. Then she looked down at the flour dusting her baby carrier.

"That wasn't my fault," she said. "Besides, Rolf saved my life."

Waman took a step forward.

"A child is not yours to sacrifice when you need a problem solved, Lenore," he said, taking another step forward. "A child is not a bargaining chip, a political tool, a scapegoat, or a weapon for one parent to use against another. A child isn't a hobby, a distraction, a plaything, a pet or a toy." His voice was rising with fury and intensity as he edged closer, driving her back against the Flippy Frog stall. "And above all, a child is not to be taken for granted!"

He was now trembling with fury.

"I didn't take it for granted, Professor Waman, honestly."

He slapped her across the face.

"A child is NEVER an 'it,' Lenore. It is a 'he.' Or a 'she.' He or she are persons, persons to be loved, cared for and fought *for*, not to be fought over."

His hand closed around her throat.

"My real mother was taken from me. I thought my new home would be the answer to my prayers and dreams." He had not begun to squeeze yet, but Lenore couldn't move or fight back. "Instead, I entered a broken home, my parents separated, fighting all the time. She carried on constant affairs with whomever she pleased. He drugged her, made a fool of her. And in the middle of it was a small, innocent child."

He raised his free hand into a tense claw.

"These hands, these arms, which should have been used to embrace his parents with love, were instead used by them as the rope in a cruel tug-of-war."

"Professor Waman . . . please . . ." All the rage and strength she had used to fight Dimitri had fled.

"I'm more than a professor, Lenore," he said ominously. "I am *this!*"

A moment later he had changed.

"I am your death!"

The hand around her neck doubled in size and began to squeeze.

The glowing tunnel ended in a large, empty tent. When they emerged from it, B'ritnee waved her hands, and the tunnel faded away. At the same time, feeble lightbulbs flickered to life around the tent, barely fighting back the darkness. The tent was empty, save for a velvet-covered barstool in the center of the room. Buddy could smell food somewhere nearby.

"How're you doing, Old Man?" he asked.

Away from the cotton candy cart, the Old Man

seemed lost and confused. He just shook his head as he gazed warily around the tent. Buddy patted him on the shoulder.

"It'll be all right."

"Brion!" B'ritnee bellowed in a deep, resonant voice. She stood next to the stool, her hands in the air, calling out to the sky in a voice that echoed eerily. "Oberon! Come to me!"

Buddy pulled the Old Man close. He half expected the roof of the tent to tear open and a great demon answer the summons.

As it turned out, he was half right.

Beyond the far door of the tent he could sense movement. Then a voice answered B'ritnee's call.

"I'm coming, I'm coming." The man's voice sounded irritated.

Just then half a man came into view in the passageway. Buddy had seen pictures of old circus freaks that looked like this, but he'd never seen one in person. Strange orange globes circled the creature. When he came to the doorway, the sight of B'ritnee made him stop.

"Oh, Iguanita," he said, looking like he was suppressing a laugh. "What a brilliant costume. Playing with the children, I presume?"

With the suppressed smile stuck on his face, he padded on his hands over to his stool and climbed up nimbly.

"I thought I had lost you," he told B'ritnee. "But now you're back, calling me by the Old Name, so it must be important." B'ritnee opened her mouth to speak, but the half-man ignored her and looked over at Buddy. "Hello there. I am Brion."

Buddy started to introduce himself, but he saw B'ritnee fuming at the slight.

"Brion!" she called out. "What issss going on here? I found purple cotton candy! That issss the dark magic. We don't ussse the dark magic."

"You're right, we don't," he answered patiently. "But he does."

"Who?" she asked. A look of shock appeared on her face, and she answered her own question. "My sssson? My sssson issss here?"

"*Our* son," Brion said, his tone a gentle rebuke. "That's one of the reasons he ran off in the first place. Anyway, surprise!"

"Where issss he?" B'ritnee rushed frantically at Brion. She shook him by the shoulders, threatening to knock him from the chair. "Where issss our sssson?"

Brion wrapped his own arms around her. This steadied him and seemed to calm her down.

"He's in the Midway, my dear," he answered. Almost as an afterthought, he added, "I believe he's about to murder someone."

23

The creature wasn't just strangling her, it was crushing her throat. Slowly. This spurred Lenore into action once more. With one hand, she tried to pry the viselike fingers from her. She knew the effort was futile, but it provided cover for her right hand as it searched the counter for anything she could use as a weapon. Finally, one of her hands closed against a frog-a-pult. Resting only on a pin upon which it rotated, the heavy metal launcher lifted easily from its base. She brought it up at the beast and connected solidly with its nose.

The creature staggered backwards. Choking, fighting for breath, Lenore pulled herself over the counter. The creature that had been Professor Waman slashed blindly at her leg as she tumbled over, but it missed. A pile of rubber frogs just behind the counter broke her fall.

"You require a slow, more painful death," it bellowed. "I am happy to oblige."

She crawled quickly on her hands and knees to the opposite side of the stall. Behind her, wood splintered as the creature tore through the counter to get to her. As she'd expected, fleeing into the stall seemed to be buying her more time than if she had just tried to run off over open ground. The creature was too big to squeeze comfortably into the stall and would have to tear it apart to get to her.

But what was she buying time for? Time to figure out how to fight the creature? Or time to say her prayers before the creature tucked her into bed permanently?

The beast stood and roared. Cords suspending stuffed animals tangled in its horns. It roared again as it tore them from its face, then ripped apart the roof itself, tearing it into pieces and flinging it away. Stuffing from shredded plush toys filled the air like dogwood fluff.

The beast tore the lily pad table loose from its base and tossed it across the Midway. It flew like a Frisbee and destroyed the Free Throw booth.

He would be upon her in moments. Unless she did something, her stalling tactic would have only served to delay her death. And piss him off even more. Given her hope not to die painfully, she had to come up with something. Looking down at her chest, a glimmer of an idea winked to life in her brain.

Lenore unstrapped the chest carrier. Squeezing the flour bag, she found that Rolf had lost less than a quarter of its contents. Excellent. Grasping the top set of carrier straps in one fist, she cradled Rolf in her arms like a child. Standing slowly, she hummed to herself.

"You offer yourself to me, do you?" said the beast. She stood just out of reach of his claws.

"Sssshhh!" she told him, raising a finger to her lips. "You'll wake the baby."

"It is too late for that," it said, but it stopped moving forward.

Lenore's humming turned into a song. She gently rocked Rolf in her arms.

"Rock-a-bye baby, on the treetop," she sang. "When the wind blows, the cradle will rock. When the wind blows, the cradle will fall. And up will go baby, cradle and all."

She didn't look up at the creature, but she could tell he had still not moved. What's more, he had fallen silent.

"That was beautiful," he said quietly. "I haven't been sung to in ages. But the word is 'down.' 'Down will come baby.' "

"No, 'up,' " she said evenly, finally looking into the creature's face, her own expression blank. "As in 'up yours!' "

Moving too fast for the beast to react, Lenore swung the child carrier on its straps like a slingshot. Like a postmodern David, she let the carrier fly right at the beast. Rolf exploded against his face, blinding him. Flour bloomed into a dense cloud around him, denser than the fog, and clung to his eyes and nose. He was blinded and choking. As an added bonus, the bag itself became impaled on his horns, leaving him clawing at his own face, roaring.

Lenore leaped over the debris of the Flippy Frog booth and ran to Zander. Fishing in his pocket, she pulled out the car keys she knew would be there.

"Yes!" she said, pumping the air instinctively. If she was lucky, she could lose herself in the fog long enough to make her way back to Zander's Kharmann Ghia. Then she would head straight for the police.

She turned to make a break for it, but a giant clawed hand closed around her neck. She was hoisted up into the air, choking. She grabbed the thickly muscled arm before her so that her neck wouldn't break outright.

"Nice try," said the beast. "Try singing a lullaby now."

Lenore kicked at him, but he held her too far out. The black fireworks returned.

Just then a white-and-tan blur rocketed from out of the fog, hitting the beast in the midsection. It dropped Lenore immediately.

Choking and sputtering, she lay on the ground, watching two blurry figures struggle before her.

"You!" bellowed the creature, who then lifted the attacker into the air and threw him across the Midway. He landed in a booth with a crash, followed by the sound of water spraying.

Lenore staggered to her feet and rubbed her eyes. For the moment, the creature, only a dark blotch in her vision, had forgotten about her. It thundered toward the game stall. Then her eyes cleared.

The Water Racers apparatus had been destroyed. The ground around it had become a muddy swamp. And lying amid the destruction was a familiar figure.

"Professor Waman?" she whispered.

Just as the creature reached the prone figure of her professor, the man came to life, kicking at the beast's chest. The force launched the creature up and over Lenore. It landed on the Bottle Ring Toss booth, smashing it with the sound of a thousand exploding chandeliers.

Professor Waman—or the superpower version of him, based on what Lenore had witnessed—leaped to his feet and marched toward the Bottle Ring Toss booth. A tinkling of glass from within indicated that the creature was moving. And then, the beast burst from the booth, glass and canvas flying everywhere. He ran at Waman, head down, ready to impale the professor on his horns.

Instead of dodging, Waman lowered his head and charged forward.

The two met with a deafening crack. A bright orange light flared around them, and both were thrown backwards. Impossibly, both remained on their feet, swaying like punch-drunk boxers.

Shaking it off, they prepared for a second charge.

"STOP!!" boomed a disembodied voice, which seemed to come from everywhere and nowhere at the same time.

The combatants froze. Waman looked triumphant; the creature, fearful.

Three orange balls of light materialized between the two. From them, three figures emerged.

"That. Is. Enough," said a very short man with a deep voice. Lenore did a double take when she realized that the man wasn't simply short, but even his deformity didn't distract her from the certainty that, though he was the smallest one present, he was the most powerful.

At the half-man's side stood a young couple. She recognized one of them from campus as the leader of a mediocre barbershop octet. He just looked around with a dopey grin, as if he had just gotten off the most rad roller coaster ride ever. The other, a blond girl about her own age, she had never seen before. In her eyes, Lenore saw that the girl was more than a student and, perhaps, more than human. At the sight of Professor Waman, who was clearly twice her age, the girl's face lit up.

"My son!" she cried and flung her arms around the man.

Waman awkwardly returned the hug. The half-man just nodded, half sad, half amused. Then he called over to Lenore.

"Come here, child. My name is Brion. The danger is over."

"It's cool," the Globe student assured her. She approached the strange group and stood beside the student, who introduced himself as Buddy.

"Mother?"

This voice came from behind the girl. From the creature.

The girl froze in the midst of lavishing an increasingly uncomfortable Waman with kisses. She turned to look at the creature.

"Ajit?" she asked. "Why do you look like Puck?"

The creature crossed his hands, growling. "Leave me alone," it said.

"That thing tried to kill me!" Lenore wasn't sure what she was witnessing, but she wanted to make sure all the facts were laid out.

"Is that true?" the blond girl asked.

"Of course it is, Mother," the creature roared, turning suddenly. "But don't think that just because you let me have my fun that I'm coming back."

"What are you talking about, Ajit?" she asked. "I didn't even know you were here." She thought for a moment, then turned to the half-man.

"Brion?" she asked, tapping her foot.

"Figures he'd trick you," said the creature. "Some things never change."

"Now, son—," Oberon began.

"I'm not your son!" the creature roared.

"Let's not start that," Oberon snapped. "We are a family, if you would just care to join it."

"You call us a family? You always made it abundantly clear that you preferred an employee to a son."

Then he turned to the blond girl. "And you, with your dalliances."

The girl blushed but said nothing.

"Dear boy," the girl said, taking his large claw in her delicate white hand. "We travel together now. And everything that troubles you happened so long ago, centuries. In one night in the woods. No one got hurt."

"What about me?" said the creature in an injured tone. But he did not pull away from the girl.

Oberon padded up to them. "Look, we are not perfect. And feel free to blame us for some of how you feel. But really, Ajit, it has been several centuries since you ran off. How much are you to blame for how you feel after all this time away?" He joined hands with the girl and the creature. "And even so, are any of these humans to blame for how you feel? For the wrongs you believe we have done to you?"

"I have been trying to help," he snarled. "I became a professor to save people from my fate!"

"And by help, you mean killing them?"

The sharp rebuke started to raise the hackles on the creature's back. Lenore was afraid the scene would erupt in violence once more. Out of the corner of her eye, she could see Professor Waman tense. Only the Globe student seemed unconcerned. He was so riveted by the bizarre scene that the only thing he seemed to be missing was popcorn.

"And poor Puck," Brion continued. "Trapping him

the only way a creature of nature can be imprisoned, in a cocoon of artificial materials. Not to mention trapping him in your form and you taking his."

The figure that resembled Professor Waman growled but said nothing. Lenore thought he looked a little embarrassed as well.

"You tried," Brion assured Waman. "We cannot always prevail, especially against such rage and sadness."

"Puck couldn't capture me himself, so you lured me here with the promise of the massacre?" said the creature. "I appreciate the effort, and I certainly accomplished what I was after, but that won't make me stay."

"You are free to go," Brion said.

"Hey, wait!" said Lenore, remembering the tent full of dead students. "He's killed many people, tried to kill me. You can't just let him go."

"I cannot force him to stay, despite what I have done to win him back," he told her. Then he gave her a sly wink and turned back to the creature. "At least stay for the banquet tonight, my son."

"What banquet?" it asked, immediately suspicious.

"This is what I've been trying to tell you. Tonight your mother and I celebrate our wedding anniversary. We only wish you to join us tonight, then you are free. This seemed to be the only way to bring you here."

"Your anniversary?" said the creature, slapping a hand to his forehead. "I had forgotten." He turned to the girl. "Mother, did you know about this?"

"Not at all," she answered. "I sssstopped hoping for your return decadessss ago. It lookssss like your father issss indeed up to hissss old trickssss."

"Bringing you back into the family seemed like the best present I could give to your mother," he told the creature. "Is that so wrong? But as I said, I can only invite you to join us, I cannot make you stay."

"Very clever, Brion," the girl said. "Disssstracting me with the ssssurprisssse of hiring a boy band so that I didn't see the *real* ssssurprisssse. I thank you." Turning to the creature, she said, "Will you pleassse come home? I missss my sssson."

"I do too," Brion added.

The creature lowered his head and thought for a moment. He raised it, not smiling.

"All right," he said. "But then you'll leave me alone."

"It is all we can ask!" said Brion. He clapped his hands together. "There are still a few more preparations."

He turned to Buddy. "You must now join your friends and prepare yourselves for your performance. Will that do?"

"Spiff-i-riffic, Mr. Brion," Buddy said.

"Excellent. Apparently, your friends have gotten along quite well with our kind. It's too bad you were led astray." He looked up at the girl and winked.

"Not at all, sir," Buddy replied. "B'ritnee was a true lady."

"That she is, son, that she is." Turning to the creature, the girl and Waman, he said, "We can't have our ceremony with anyone in false guises, so let us stop first at the Magick Mirror Maze."

"It's all right, Father," said the creature. Oberon glowed with pride at the sound of being called Father. "I don't need to go."

He reverted to his Professor Waman form before them.

"I've learned much while I've been on my own in the world," he said, with not a small amount of pride.

"Like the dark magic of purple cotton candy?" said the girl, displeasure in her voice. He just squirmed under her glare.

"Is that how you really look?" Lenore asked. The man was relieved for the subject change.

"Indeed. My name really is Ajit Waman," he said. "And I really am a college professor. The gentleman there, his name is Puck." The Waman who had saved Lenore bowed his head to her.

"So he looks like a big horned thing?"

"Indeed. Wouldn't harm a fly, though," Waman said. "Except in extreme cases, as this case warranted. Anyway, I always thought such a fearsome visage was wasted on such a gentle soul, so I appropriated it."

"I see."

"Do you forgive me, gentle Puck?" Waman said to his double, who only grunted in reply.

"Sadly, he hasn't spoken in centuries," he told Lenore. "Sad. His tongue used to be the cleverest thing about him."

"Follow me, everyone," Oberon told them. "Stay close. I have unbound the fog, but you can still trip on something if you're not careful."

"What about the others?" Lenore asked. Her friends remained unconscious not far away.

"I'll send others for them," he said. "Fear not. They will come to no further harm."

With that, he led the group away from the Midway, walking before them on his hands.

24

During their short walk, Lenore could feel a tremendous change in the atmosphere of the place. The fog no longer seemed to cling to her. The feeling of a cliff hidden just ahead subsided.

It just seemed like fog.

"What did you mean when you said you'd 'unbound' the fog?" Lenore asked.

"A spell," he told her. "A magic by which we could keep everyone, especially my son, within the confines of the park."

"But all the people he killed?"

Oberon motioned for the group to stop and rested his torso on the ground. He reached a hand to hers.

"Our ways are strange and unfathomable, young one," he said. "Suffice it to say, the prospect of a wholesale slaughter was the lure for our son. And the fog was the means to keep him here once he got here."

"That's monstrous!" she cried, pulling away from him. "All those people, in that tent! Just so you could reunite with your son!" The image of Murph and Polly, their agonized faces floating in the darkness, rose in her memory. "You're horrible. More than horrible!"

"As I say, our ways are not the ways of man," he said in a patient, kindly voice. "And by the end of this evening, perhaps things will not be so bad, even if you cannot find it in your heart to forgive us."

Lenore was torn by his soothing words and the horror of what she had seen in the banquet room. Before she could sort out her feelings, the group stood before the Magick Mirror Maze.

"Here we are," said Brion. He gestured toward the entrance. "Iguanita, Puck, if you please."

Puck entered the maze immediately. Lenore saw a bright flash of orange, and he disappeared. Before Iguanita entered, she approached Buddy and took his hands.

"Your grandmother was right, you know," she told him. "Some mazes show you who you really are."

"But you said it depended on which side you entered?"

"Yes," she said. "I want to prepare you. Earlier in the evening, I entered the maze through the exit."

He paused for a second and thought. "So . . . you look how you *wanted* to look, not how you really look, right?"

"Exactly," she said. "I'm going to go in the front now, and when I return, I'll look like the real me. I hope you'll forgive the deception and not find me hideous."

"Hey," he said with a wink, lightly cuffing her chin with one hand and pressing the other to his heart. "The beauty's in here."

She kissed him lightly on the forehead and entered the maze. Buddy continued to watch, as if bidding farewell to a great love. Another flash of orange light and she was gone.

Buddy turned to the other and let out a great sigh.

"This is gonna freak me out, isn't it?" he gasped.

Waman laughed and clapped him on the shoulder. Likewise amused, Brion motioned for the others to follow them around to the back of the Mirror Maze. It didn't take long for them to see orange light within the maze, pulsing brighter and brighter.

"It's an incremental process," Waman explained. "Each mirror changes you a bit."

Finally, a flash emitted from the exit and a tall figure emerged.

Lenore took a step back. It was the creature that had tried to kill her.

Seeing her apprehension, the creature—Puck, she tried hard to remind herself—hunched itself to appear smaller. He smiled, and the fangs in his mouth suddenly looked silly, not frightening. Lenore smiled back. Puck reached out his hand, and she responded likewise. His touch was warm and gentle. Looking into his eyes, she found no malice whatsoever. He could have been a child in a Halloween costume.

The entrance flashed again and another figure emerged. Buddy's jaw dropped open.

B'ritnee had been replaced by a large woman who appeared to be part lizard. She looked at Buddy, then quickly looked away.

"Ah, there's my Iguanita," Brion said. "As radiant as my Titania ever was."

She smiled to acknowledge the compliment, but she still couldn't face Buddy. Lenore could see why. He was, after all, a normal, attractive human. And she had "dressed up" in human clothes. Buddy's reaction was hard to gauge. Then a huge grin spread across his face.

"You didn't say you were a hot lizard chick, B'ritnee!" he said.

"It's Iguanita," she replied, her colors cycling in embarrassment.

"Just as well. B'ritnee's a dumb name anyway." He stepped forward and took her by the hands. "And don't worry, the real B'ritnees I know aren't any less fake than what you were. At least your alterations come for free. They have to pay for beauty like that."

Iguanita's colors settled into a slow rhythm. Her neckfin relaxed, and she looked into his eyes.

"At least you're the real thing," he continued, "one hundred percent, genuine lizard skin. I don't know whether to marry you or accessorize with you."

"That'ssss no way to sssspeak to a queen!" She tried to act serious and offended, but she couldn't help giggling. She looked down again, her colors falling into a deep pink shade.

"You cannot marry her, son," said a good-natured Brion. "She's taken. Come now, let us begin the celebration!"

The banquet overwhelmed every sense Lenore possessed. She and Buddy were invited to sit near the head of an impossibly long table with Brion, Oberon, Puck and Ajit.

"Is it me," asked Lenore, "or is this tent bigger on the inside than it is on the outside?"

"It's not just you," Buddy answered. "I think it's another show of our host's mojo."

Around them, a multitude of strange creatures mingled with humans. She saw something that looked like a werewolf and a blond woman with a snake's body that had been introduced as Serpentina. Next to her sat a pinheaded man. She recognized him as Tip-Tip from his housecoat. Sitting among the Perpetuals were students from Globe, members of Buddy's boy band, who chatted like old friends. One boy, a particularly pale-looking freshman, seemed to be getting quite cozy with a girl with the slimy, maroon, ridged skin of a worm.

Lenore started at the sight of Violet Eyes and Ass-Face among the revelers. They and other elderly guests, all local homeless Stratford residents, as well as

Buddy's friend, the Old Man, seemed at ease, conversing and rubbing elbows with humans and Perpetuals alike.

In all, there were several dozen creatures and humans. They spoke in English, foreign tongues, inhuman language, as well as in an assortment of animal sounds and Tip-Tip's gibberish. It all blended in a low, pleasant roar.

Before each reveler were set plates piled high with meats, vegetables and fruits of all kinds. Baskets filled with fresh, warm bread, steam rising from it, sat every few feet. Each place setting included cups of homemade beer and wine, as well as crystal-clear water and freshly squeezed juices; none could be lifted without spilling some, they were filled so closely to the top.

The smells were so distinct and fresh, so vivid, that her mind perceived them as colors and emotions. But even that did not prepare her for the taste. Each bite was an explosion of sweetness and savory, hearty full flavors delivered with a full palette of textures, from smooth sauces to the coarse grains on the bread crusts.

Lenore speared a tender slice of meat from her plate and lifted it to her mouth. Suddenly, the image of her classmates, their bodies lying in the room, rose in her mind. She remembered the strong smells rising from the pots on the table. She put it together: the setup reminded her of a smokehouse.

She gagged, dropping her fork. It clattered onto her plate.

"Is something the matter?" asked Brion. The room had fallen quiet, and all eyes were on her.

"No. Yes. This meat." She pointed down to her plate. "What is it?"

She became aware that of her classmates, only Rosenberg and Gyllenhal sat at the table. They were across from her. Rosenberg wiped a spot of food from Pete Gyllenhal's face while the two listened.

"It's beef," Brion said, mystified. After a moment, he seemed to understand her concern and added, "We purchased it honestly, and did not steal any of your local cattle, I promise you."

"No," she said, choking on her words. "The others. I saw them. In a tent. It looked like they were being . . . cured and seasoned."

Brion frowned, trying hard to figure out what she was talking about. Then his eyebrows went up and he burst out laughing. Others around him joined in, not even sure what they were laughing at.

"You think we've cooked your friends?" he gasped out. "Oh, dear child!" He turned to Iguanita. "She thinks we're eating her friends!"

The entire room erupted in laughter, particularly the Perpetuals, who seemed in on the joke. Lenore squirmed in her seat, the infectious laughter fighting the horror of her suspicions.

"I assure you this is beef, my child," Brion told her, fighting hard to calm himself. "And you are half-right.

They *were* being cured. But not in the way you mean. I give you my word."

"But they were dead . . . murdered . . ." She glanced at Ajit, who gave her an apologetic smile.

"Such dark words at such a light occasion," Brion said. "Fear not. All will be mended. Please enjoy your meal. Tasty as it is, it is quite an ordinary meal."

"What about Dimitri and the others?" Lenore asked.

"They are resting, dear. You will see them after the celebration."

Brion signaled for the dinner to resume. Everyone turned immediately back to their plates and their conversations.

Lenore poked hesitantly at her plate for a few moments. She wanted to trust Brion, but she still felt uncomfortable. Then she lifted her fork and brought it to her mouth once more. And she took a bite. Her taste buds immediately maxed out on the succulent meat, herbed to perfection. After that, it was all Lenore could do to eat politely, using utensils, rather than to greedily stuff fistfuls of food into her mouth like a Viking.

Across the table, Gyllenhal shoveled forkloads of food into his face as if it were his last meal. Both he and Rosenberg still wore their baby carriers on their chests.

"Kina annoying, isn't it?" Waman said, touching her shoulder, looking in the couple's direction. "Those two came equipped enough to survive in case a nuclear war broke out while they were strolling around the carnival," he said, shaking his head in amusement. "Spent most of the time searching the park for a baby-changing station. They're the only ones who truly deserve a passing grade."

The rest of the dinner passed with a constant flow of amiable chatter, plates that seemed to fill themselves up with food and bottomless cups of refreshment. Appreciative belches punctuated the proceedings, and when it was over, Lenore herself let one rip, much to the delight of the crowd.

Finally, Brion clapped his hands twice to gain the room's attention. As they quieted down, he cleared a space on the table before him and hopped onto it from his stool. He held up a cup of wine.

"My friends, old and new, I thank you for sharing this evening with me and my queen, Iguanita. This has been a trying night for all, some more than others." He gravely toasted Lenore. "But the perceived horrors of the evening were only to ensure that a greater joy infuse our celebration. We have been reunited at last with our son." He lifted his cup to Ajit, who returned the toast. "We have made new friends," he said, indicating the students and other human guests, "and most of all, I am able to profess, before all of you, my love for my wife, Iguanita, queen of the Perpetuals. Though the world has moved on from us, we have remained together. And together we will remain, forever."

He lifted his cup to the entire room, bidding the rest of the gathering to join him. They did, and after a raucous toast, everyone drank deeply.

Oberon raised his hands to silence the cheering and whistling that broke out after the toast.

"And now, I have arranged for a talented group of musicians to entertain us." He turned toward Buddy. "Are you and your fellows ready, Master Bragg?"

"Righteously!" Buddy said and stood.

"Excellent! My friends, my dear wife, I present to you The Shower Tones!"

Buddy gathered the group at the edge of the tent. He stood center, flanked by the rest of The Shower Tones, their backs to the audience. The table fell completely still. Buddy gave the guys a thumbs-up, then hummed a note. Flutie and Thomas followed that with a dueling beat box introduction as the rest of them moved up and down in rhythm, turning toward the audience one by one. When they were all facing forward, Buddy led them through their sexy interpretation of "Coney Island Baby."

About midway through, as they were performing a synchronized hip gyration, the hooting started. The female Perpetuals, particularly the ones who had been sitting next to the group's members, became particularly vocal. The girl who looked like a worm called out Trevin's name in glee, causing the freshman to blush. But he didn't miss a beat or a note. The Pinhead got into the act and hopped up in his place, singing along in gibberish. Iguanita's colors pulsed to the beat of the music. Buddy noticed that even the humans seemed to be caught up in the music.

Tonight was indeed a night of firsts.

Then came the big finish, and The Shower Tones tore their shirts open. Worm girl screamed out Trevin's name once more and fainted. Serpentina shed an entire layer of skin out of excitement. Iguanita led the room in thunderous applause.

"Encore!" Iguanita cried. "Please, again!"

The group looked to Buddy. Even he was surprised at the request.

"Why the hell not?" he said to them and started to snap his shirt. The rest followed suit. "One more time!" he called out.

"With the smoothness!" seconded the bass singer named Johnson.

They turned their backs to the crowd, and within seconds launched into their second set of beat boxing, hip gyrations and sexy synchronized come-ons.

The second time around, Tip-Tip joined them before the crowd, tearing his housecoat open at the end, sending most of the audience falling from their chairs in hysterics.

25

After The Shower Tones' third encore, the exhausted performers nearly collapsed into their seats. They were immediately thronged by fans among the Perpetuals.

Soon after, the tables were cleared and removed from the tent, and chairs were pushed against the tent wall. Someone set up a Victrola, its horn bellowing out scratchy, slow tunes from a vinyl record.

Lenore watched The Shower Tones and Perpetuals interact. Wes, one of the group's tenors, was getting very chummy with Hermaphrodite. The Worm Girl clung to her idol, Trevin, like Lycra.

Good for them, she thought. Happy ending for them. But despite Brion's assurances, the image of the dead students continued to haunt her.

"You look troubled, my dear," Brion said, padding up to her. "Come, dance with me."

"Um, how do we dance?" Lenore asked.

"Here. Let me put my arm around you," Oberon said. "I'll hang on to your shoulders. Don't worry, I'm really quite light."

And he was, surprisingly so for how solidly his upper body appeared to be built. She easily carried him to the center of the dance floor. His hands felt rough and thickly callused against hers.

"Thank you, my dear," Brion said after they had silently made a couple of slow turns. "At least I am not troubled with two left feet!"

Lenore smiled, but clearly Brion was looking for more of a reaction.

"The deaths are weighing heavily upon you, aren't they?" he asked.

"Of course," she said. "Shouldn't Ajit pay for what he's done?"

"Well, let me ask this," Oberon said. "What if the damage he had wrought could be undone?"

"I wish."

"We used to be fairies, you know."

"Like in the books? With butterfly wings?" Lenore asked.

Brion chuckled. "Yes, something like that. Once upon a time we gamboled in forests, played pranks in villages and brought together lovers." His eyes seemed to mist at the memory. "We were beauty incarnate."

"What happened?"

"Part of it is that humans stopped believing in us.

Though we retain our powers, our physical forms have slowly mutated as the world has moved on and lost its innocence, as its belief in nature's creatures fades."

Lenore's face grew hot with emotion.

"Feel not sad for us, my dear," Oberon told her, catching a tear that rolled down her cheek. "We remain, we endure. That is why we call ourselves the Perpetuals now. You may not always see us, and in many ways, you may not wish to see us, but we are always here."

"But why do you keep yourselves a secret?" she asked. "If you worked openly, performed your miracles, you would give humans a reason to believe."

Oberon laughed bitterly. "Then we would truly become a freak show," he said. "And besides, that humanity stopped believing in us was only part of the problem."

"What's the other part?"

Brion rested his head on her shoulder and sighed heavily. It was the sound of centuries of weariness.

"We stopped believing in humanity," he said. He fell silent, his face sad. Then he made an effort to smile. "As I have said, heavy words on such a joyous occasion. We will bring back to life all of Surg's victims."

"That's over a hundred people! Fairies have that kind of power?"

"Not always," he told her. "Except for tonight. We are creatures of life and nature. An anniversary celebration is a celebration of life. Better still, it is a celebration that connects the past to the future. And so tonight, according to our custom, we have the power to return the future to those any of our kind have deprived of it."

They danced together in silence until the record began skipping at its center. Around them, the celebration was winding down. In one corner of the tent, a group comprised of Shower Tones and their Perpetual fans huddled around Buddy and Iguanita. They spoke passionately in low voices. The Shower Tones seemed to be begging a favor of the queen. She seemed to agree to something, and a few of them hopped up and down in place, excited. Serpentina slithered around Thomas, one of the bass singers, coiling at his waist.

Buddy and Iguanita detached from the group, with two of The Shower Tones close behind.

"Set me down on the table, dear," Brion asked Lenore as the small group approached.

"I have a request from our human friends, Brion," she said.

"Totally," Buddy said. "Seems we've got some real love connections going on here."

"Is that so?" asked Brion.

Wes spoke up. "That Hermaphrodite. Got it going on in more ways than one, you know what I mean?"

"And . . . and . . . Earthworm Evelyn really likes me," stammered Trevin. "I don't feel, like, so nervous around her."

"Isn't Evelyn involved with the Human Armadillo?" Brion was taken aback by Trevin's suggestion.

"No, no, it's not like that, I swear," he said quickly. "She said she would break herself in half and I could, like, you know, date her other half."

"I see," Brion said. His brow creased deeply in contemplation. "Iguanita, my sweet, have the humans been informed that to remain with us, they will need to shed their human forms?"

"Yes, I told them, Brion," she answered, turning to Buddy.

"They're down with it, sir," he said.

"Totally down," Wes said.

"Yes, please, sir," Trevin chirped.

Brion thought a moment longer, then addressed the room.

"I give my consent for the humans to join us! Take them down Magick Mirror Maze so that their true forms may be revealed!"

The Shower Tones and their Perpetual paramours erupted in cheers and hugs of joy.

Together, the group marched to the maze entrance. One by one, Brion laid a hand on the head of each Shower Tone. With evident trepidation, Quincy entered first. An orange light flashed, and he was gone. He was followed by Flutie, who gave a thumbs-up before he went in.

"Maybe I'll come out looking like Luther," Thomas joked as he entered.

Trevin practically ran into the Mirror Maze, anxious to be with his clone of Earthworm Evelyn.

Ty examined the doorway closely. "Here goes nothing." And he was gone.

Uni bowed several times before Brion and Iguanita. He even bowed to Buddy and Lenore. "Thank you. Thank you. Very honored. Thank you."

Wes entered last, with his characteristic saunter.

"What about you, Buddy?" asked Lenore after the last of his group had walked to the maze's exit.

"Nah, that's not the life for me," he said. "If I left, who else would care for Globe's inevitable Cavalcade of Oddities, aka geeky freshmen?"

Lenore rolled his statement over in her mind as they waited for The Shower Tones to emerge from the Magick Mirror Maze. Quincy came out first, sporting eight suction-cup-covered tentacles. Flutie's neck had stretched by several feet; he had sprouted gray plumage and walked on the powerful legs of an ostrich. Thomas strutted out, covered in dark scales. His pupils had become vertical slits in his eyes.

"Check it," he said and flared his neck into a hood like a king cobra. Long fangs completed the image. "Oh, the sssssmoothnesssss!" he hissed.

Trevin emerged, almost unrecognizable. The small, pale boy had grown by two feet and packed on at least fifty pounds of muscle, most of it on his neck, which sported a bristly Mohawk. Tusks curled up on either side of a wet, pink snout.

"I could go for some truffles," snorted the newly formed Razorback Boy.

A duckbilled creature, covered in fur, waddled out next.

"I'm a platypus?" whined Ty. "My true form is **a** platypus? Can I get a refund?"

"You have made your choice, young man," Brion told him.

"I'm only kidding, I'm cool," he said quickly. "Seriously. I've always wanted poisonous spurs." He waddled over to his newly transformed cohorts.

Uni announced himself as a voice in their heads before he stepped out of the maze.

"That was incredible, guys," he said, clearly and in perfect English.

And then he stood before them, antennae twitching above his head, sporting brown claws like those of a lobster.

"No, I'm a Crayfish Man," he said in their minds. "And no, I'm *not* speaking English, Buddy. I'm speaking directly to your mind, beyond language."

"Can you read minds too?" Buddy asked.

"Yes," they all heard. "But don't worry, Buddy, I won't tell what I just saw."

Buddy blushed and looked to the ground. Uni clicked his claws twice to demonstrate, and then he joined the rest.

Wes emerged looking exactly the same.

"I guess it didn't work for you," Buddy said.

Wes responded with a secretive smirk. "Let's just say that me and Hermaphrodite are a complete double date on Saturday night, you know what I mean?"

"For once, I wish I didn't," Buddy said with a sour expression.

"Welcome to the Perpetuals," Brion told them. "Now go, begin your new lives."

Each transformed Shower Tone shook Buddy's hand in turn, with tentacle, claw and wing. As the last one walked off, Lenore could see that Buddy's cool composure was on the verge of melting entirely.

"Your friendssss will be happy," Iguanita told him. "You brought them among ussss and that makessss you resssssponssssible for their happinessss, assss you will be for otherssss at your sssschool and all through your life."

Buddy remained speechless, watching his friends disappear in the thinning fog.

"My queen," Brion said quietly. "Please take Master Bragg to the Old Man. There is a last bit of business I must attend to with Lenore."

"Yessss." Iguanita put an arm around Buddy and led him away.

26

"What will happen to everyone?" Lenore asked once they were alone.

"By morning, this fog will lift. When it does, everyone will be restored to their former lives, including the vagrants we 'enlisted' and Mr. Bragg's elderly friend. All of Ajit's 'victims' will find themselves at home, in bed, with no memory of the events related to our little Fun Faire."

Lenore was relieved. It seemed a gargantuan task, bringing the dead back to life, but from what she had seen of Brion and the Perpetuals, she believed he could do it.

"What about Ajit? Anger like his, the killing-over-a-hundred-people-in-a-night kind of anger, doesn't blow away like fog."

"Correct," he told her. "But I am pleased to report that Ajit has agreed to stay with us for the time being. It will not be easy, but at least we are together. Most importantly, we are a family again. Both his mother and I *have* changed, and not just physically. And perhaps, in time, all wounds will be healed."

"I feel like Dorothy at the end of the Wizard of Oz," Lenore said. "Guess there's no fairy magic for me."

"Your dreams are not unknown to me, my dear," he told her.

"So you know? About Dimitri?" He nodded silently and looked away. "You said that's what fairies do, bring together lovers."

She stopped him, daring to place a hand on his shoulder.

"Can you do this for me?" she begged. "Can you?"

He searched her face, frowning. Drawing a measured breath, he asked, "Do you think everyone's dreams should come true?"

"What do you mean?"

"Just because you wish to share a life with Dimitri, is this how it should be? What of Zander's desires for you? Or Mia's for Zander?"

The intensity of Brion's expression warned Lenore not to answer hastily.

"Well, it would be helpful to Mia if Dimitri left her alone," she said slowly. "And if Zander didn't leave her for me, her feelings would be spared."

"What of Zander?" he asked. "And Dimitri, for that matter? They would be living in *your* dream, unaware of the loss of their own dreams."

"You're saying I'd be messing with their minds," she said. "And that it is unfair."

"I cannot judge such a thing," he said. "The ways of the Perpetuals are different. But I am aware of how our powers affect humans. You are an intelligent girl, and I want you to understand what you are asking of me."

He wanted to deny her Dimitri, who had occupied all her waking, and much of her sleeping, moments since his kiss. *That* to her seemed the most unfair thing of all.

"You made Buddy's dream come true!" she said. "And all of his friends' dreams, too."

"Did I?" he asked. "I merely offered an opportunity. Buddy could have chosen not to accept the invitation. But he did so. And did he *really* get what he wanted? He lost many friends tonight."

"He's used to that," she said. "He goes through freshmen like water. That's his deal."

"He has changed, my dear. How could he not, with all that he has beheld tonight? Do you not understand how he will be haunted by such memories, and feel the need to outdo himself?" Brion shook his head. "Buddy will have a difficult time, for the real world does not offer such profound pleasures. To regain his dream, he will need to forget that he lived it."

"At least his friends are happy," Lenore pointed out.

"Of course they are. Now. But the time will come when they will miss their old lives, and their families and friends. Their path is irrevocable. Should they thank or curse Buddy for steering them onto that path?"

Lenore could feel tears welling up in her eyes. Brion's words were becoming a fiercer attack than Waman's monstrous claws.

"Why are you doing this, Brion?" she sobbed. "You gave Buddy the means *and* the choice. That is all I ask."

"You accept responsibility for how your actions will affect others?"

"Absolutely."

"I mean everyone, child," he said, insisting that she think again. But Lenore was at her breaking point.

"This is between the four of us!" she said, almost shouting. "There are no others! Please, Brion. Oberon. Please. If you don't even give me the chance, I'll end up the haunted one."

He shook his head, evidently disappointed. "Very well," he said, then led her back through the Fun Faire. The fog had nearly lifted. They soon arrived at the cotton candy machine, which lay crumpled on its side. Brion opened a compartment and drew out a clean, white paper cone.

"It's broken," Lenore said.

"That machine is just for show anyway," he said and held the cone in the air. His hand glowed orange, sending waves of energy up the cone. A globular shape blossomed at the top, glowing and expanding as he muttered. Lenore could see the fluffy swirls of cotton candy. Brion stopped muttering and the glow died out, leaving a large ball of cotton candy atop the cone. It was colored a pale green. He handed the cone to her.

"Take this. Share it with your friends. Zander will love Mia, who will return his love. Likewise you will become the apple of Dimitri's eye. Unlike the others, this enchantment is permanent."

She held the cotton candy before her, examining it slowly. "If it's a love potion, you'd think it would be red."

"You don't wish to discover the effects of red cotton candy, my dear," he said darkly. "Besides, this is not a 'love potion,' as you say. It will merely fulfill your dream. Let us retrieve your friends," he added, not looking at her. "You must take them home now."

They soon reentered the warren of tents. He took her to one, where her friends lay sprawled on cots. They showed no signs of the night's violence.

"An enchantment was cast upon them," he explained, "providing them rest and healing. They will awaken at dawn, refreshed. They will have no memory of tonight's events, but will otherwise return to their normal selves."

Lenore thought this sounded more like a warning than a simple explanation. But he did not continue. Instead, he summoned other Perpetuals to carry Lenore's unconscious friends to the parking lot.

"Go now, my dear," Brion said, laying a hand upon her head. "We shall not meet again."

"Yesssss, my sssssweet," hissed Iguanita, who had appeared with Waman. "I wish you a sssssafe journey and long life."

Her expression, though kind, darkened somewhat when she saw Lenore holding the green cotton candy. She shot a look to Brion, who just shrugged to indicate some helplessness. Iguanita seemed to accept this, and the two turned away from Lenore, disappearing down the far passageway.

Waman walked with her back to the car as three pairs of Perpetuals carried the others. Lenore requested that he remain in physical form so that she could talk with her former professor.

"Why does Brion seem so agitated?" she asked him. "You've returned to the fold, The Shower Tones are starting new lives and I'm sure Buddy will be all right. The Old Man and the homeless people will be taken care of. And best of all, no one died!"

A dark cloud passed over Waman's face, but before he could answer, they arrived at Zander's Kharmann Ghia.

"Wait a sec," Lenore said, slapping her forehead. "We can't take Zander's car. No backseat." She searched for Dimitri's Mustang. "Let's take them over there, guys. Sorry 'bout that."

Among the group, only Tip-Tip chittered his irritation.

Waman didn't speak in the short walk to Dimitri's car. Lenore had forgotten their conversation; she was excited about driving the Mustang.

"Hold up," she said to the Armadillo Boy and Tip-Tip, who carried Dimitri. "I need his keys."

Trying to push away the impure thoughts that rushed into her head, she reached into Dimitri's front pocket to retrieve his car keys. She found them. And something else.

As she withdrew her hand from Dimitri's pocket, she pressed the remote button, unlocking all of his doors. While the others loaded her friends into the car, she examined the square object she had found with the keys.

She knew what it was before she opened it. And she opened it, quickly.

All air, and most sense, left her body immediately.

The box contained the most exquisite diamond ring she had ever seen. An engagement ring.

"Wow," she said.

"He was going to propose to her," Waman said, his eyes going from the ring to the cotton candy in her other hand. "Guess it's yours now."

"Not necessarily," she told him and snapped the box shut. "I'm serious. I still have some thinking to do."

Slamming car doors indicated that the Perpetuals had finished their job. Dimitri rested in the front passenger seat, with Mia and Zander in the back. Waman dismissed the others, who disappeared in balls of orange light.

"So what was with the purple cotton candy, anyway?" Lenore asked. "Was it, like, homicidal flavored, so that when they ate it, they wanted to kill us?"

"Not quite, Lenore," Waman told her, suddenly very nervous. "It projected one person's darkest dreams onto another."

Lenore thought about that for a moment. "But that means one of them secretly would have wanted to kill us."

Waman nodded. He looked so serious, but then Lenore started to laugh.

"Oh, that's a good one," she said. "You almost had me. Like either of them were murderous schizos."

"Only Mia ate the cotton candy," he said. He wasn't laughing. Her own died off shortly thereafter.

"Are you saying Dimitri? . . ." she asked.

"Not everyone survived," Waman told her quietly. "Brion can only reverse what our own people have done. He cannot revive a human murdered by another human."

"Now you're really talking crazy," Lenore said.

"Look in the trunk of the Mustang, Lenore," Waman told her.

They locked eyes. At least she could tell he was being serious, even if she thought he was seriously disturbed.

"Fine!" she said, sounding angry but feeling frightened. Using the remote, she popped the trunk and looked in. What she saw in there made her drop to her knees.

A pair of yellow rubber kitchen gloves. They were caked with white and green powder.

And a brown crust, where blood had mixed with the powders.

In her mind, she replayed that evening. Finding Ione dead. The unexpected sight of Dimitri. Her mind zoomed in on his hands, and she remembered: Though almost his entire body had been covered in powder, his hands had been spotless. Tuning up the resolution of her memory, she focused on his forearms and the abrupt line where the powder had begun on both arms.

Regaining the feeling in her legs, she stood and lifted the gloves gingerly out of the trunk. She held them before Waman as if they were covered with more blood than flour and cleanser.

"She wouldn't drop the class so he could be paired with Mia," Waman explained quietly, to Lenore's mounting horror. "He was *that* obsessed with Mia. So, he pulled on a spare set of gloves and strangled her. The other Perpetuals found the body because they had been retrieving the one-eyed vagrant at the time. Even they thought I was responsible. And it's a good thing they made that mistake."

"Why?" she asked, already knowing the answer.

"Because he would have killed you. At the time, he didn't want to. But he would have. But when you returned and there was no body, he spared you.

"I'd seen this in him," Waman continued. "That's why I gave him the purple cotton candy. It was the last thing he needed to push him over the edge. When he saw himself, his murderous desires, reflected in Mia's eyes, it broke down the few barriers left in his mind. Which was my intention at the time." He shook his head sadly. "With Mia by his side, he wanted to cement the deal by getting rid of you two."

"So he *was* himself the entire time," she said. "He really wanted to kill us. He'd already murdered Ione. He's crazy."

Lenore looked into the car at the sleeping Dimitri. He repulsed her now. And frightened her. And she didn't know what to do about it.

"Yes," Waman said, "but it doesn't have to be that way. Your dream isn't about a murderer."

She looked at Waman, not comprehending. He pointed to the cotton candy.

"Give him that, and it all goes away," he told her. "He has no memory, he falls in love with you, his murderous impulses evaporate and you live happily ever after. The fairy tale ending you have been seeking."

"And Ione?"

Waman just shook his head. As Lenore let his meaning sink in, Waman kissed her forehead.

"Be well," he said and vanished in a shower of orange sparks.

Lenore stood there for several minutes, looking from the cotton candy, to the gloves, to the ring. Unable to untangle her thoughts and emotions, she carried all three with her into the Mustang.

EPILOGUE

The weather broke the next day in Stratford. A cold front moved in, and the region looked forward to lower temperatures and humidity, plus a chance of rousing thundershowers. The dry and muggy days of summer had taken a vacation.

The students of Professor Ajit Waman's Human Sexuality 101 course awoke after the best sleep of the summer. Those who remembered enough to return to class found it cancelled. One student remarked that this was just as well. "I think the dude had issues," he said.

Besides Buddy and Lenore, only Rosenberg and Gyllenhal had been allowed to retain their memories of the previous night's events. Ajit had whispered to them that it was their reward for passing the course. The two added the experience to a book they were writing together, the first chapter detailing the events in Denmark the previous fall. They also began to research the process of adopting a child.

* * *

As Brion predicted, Buddy found himself more alone than ever. What in the real world could compare to magic, fairies, freaks and a once-in-a-lifetime royal performance? He couldn't talk openly about it and elicited more ridicule than ever when he did. In the following weeks, he almost wore himself out trying to duplicate the midsummer adventure. But then fall arrived, and along with it, a new crop of freshmen. He soon realized that his world was to them what the Perpetuals' world was to him, and reaffirmed his duty to show the misfits a good time.

By October, his greatest concern was whether he'd direct his group in experimental video projects or as mimes.

Not too long after taking to the road with the Perpetuals, some of The Shower Tones wanted to contact their families. They couldn't, Brion told them. He was gentle and sympathetic, but the news was hard to take. He explained that it wasn't just a matter of whether or not their families and friends would recognize them; the magic that made them Perpetuals meant they'd never existed as humans. They had no families. They had no friends. Except for other Perpetuals.

Brion explained to them that time would soothe their newly immortal souls. And it did. But most of The

Shower Tones agreed: the first couple of centuries were hard.

All of Stratford's vagrants—Audra, Violet Eyes, Ass-Face among them—found themselves rested, nourished and wearing new clothes for the first time in years. And the pockets of the new clothes were filled with money. Brion may have kidnapped his so-called volunteers and controlled their minds, but he'd paid them well. Many used their earnings to buy alcohol. But not all. Violet Eyes, whose name was Gerome Farber, found work as a cashier in a store, the very steps of which he used to sleep on at night. Within, his boss's wife threw herself at him, and he went with it. Audra Billingsley, a former prostitute who'd possessed only the last shreds of a drug- and isolation-addled mind when the Perpetuals had "recruited" her, left the streets almost immediately. Within two years, she had a job as an executive assistant. Within five years, she had become a self-help guru. The sunglasses became her trademark. "The future's so bright, I have to wear shades!" became her slogan.

The Old Man woke up the morning after the Fun Faire left Stratford, trying to hold onto a dream about his dead wife. His pillow was wet. He hadn't even cried when she'd died. Then he wondered why his car was across his property.

"Damn fool kids," he muttered to himself as he hiked out to retrieve it.

The site of the Fun Faire was empty by morning. No one knew it had even been there. Even the grass where tents had stood, where people had walked, remained unbent.

As Midsummer Night ended, Lenore was finding it difficult to remain under the speed limit as she drove from the Fun Faire. Even though the night had become chilly, she opened both front windows. The cold sting of the air kept her alert. The others continued to sleep, Dimitri snoring in the front passenger seat, Zander tangled with Mia in the back.

Lenore looked from them to her lap, where the dish gloves Dimitri had used to murder Ione sat next to the cone of green cotton candy. She had opened the ring box so she could watch the stone glitter as she drove. She would never wear it.

Dimitri was a murderer. And if she used the magic, he would never pay for Ione's death. Lenore couldn't bear to live with such knowledge. Ione didn't deserve to be denied justice. And so Lenore made up her mind: She would drop Mia and Zander at home and present Dimitri and the gloves to the police. It was the only way for her to find peace. And perhaps, in some way, give peace to Ione.

But first, the cotton candy.

Lenore lifted the cone from her lap, ready to toss it out the window. At that moment, the car hit a rough section of road, setting the car rattling. The ring box rode the vibrations across the dashboard and hopped into Lenore's lap when the car hit a bump moments later. The ring, shaken loose from its card, fell between Lenore's thighs. Putting down the cotton candy, she fished it out of her crotch.

For the first time, she touched the ring. The smooth platinum at her fingertips dazzled her anew. Trying to keep her eyes on the road, she used her thumb and pinky to slip it onto the ring finger of her right hand.

It fit perfectly.

The diamond glittered in Lenore's eyes as she picked up the yellow rubber gloves, coated with cleanser and flour, crusted with Ione's blood, and tossed them out the car window.

Visit
❖ Pocket Books ❖
online at

....

www.SimonSays.com

....

Keep up on the latest new
releases from your favorite
authors, as well as author
appearances, news, chats,
special offers and more.

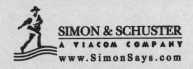

SIMON & SCHUSTER
A VIACOM COMPANY
www.SimonSays.com

Pocket
Books

2381-01